Biodynamic

CRANIOSACRAL THERAPY

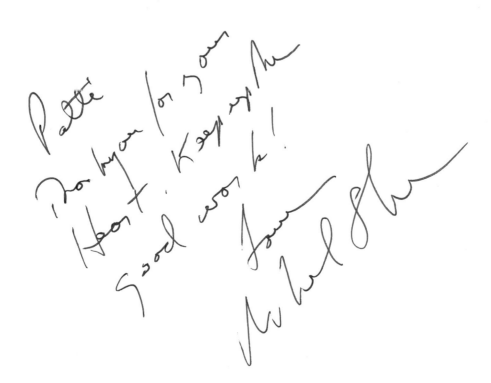

Other books by Michael Shea

Biodynamic Craniosacral Therapy, Volume One
Biodynamic Craniosacral Therapy, Volume Two
Biodynamic Craniosacral Therapy, Volume Three

Biodynamic
CRANIOSACRAL THERAPY

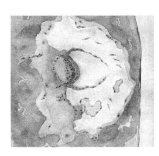

VOLUME FOUR

Michael J. Shea, PhD

With contributions from

Carol Agneessens, MS
Claudine Laabs
Sheila Shea, MA
Friedrich Wolf

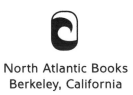

North Atlantic Books
Berkeley, California

Published by	Cover art by Friedrich Wolf
North Atlantic Books	Cover and book design by Jan Camp
P.O. Box 12327	Production by Larry Van Dyke
Berkeley, California 94712	Printed in the United States of America

All photographs in the Acknowledgments and in Chapters 13, 14, 15, 16, and 19 used with permission from the photographer, Claudine Laabs. Photographs in figures 17.14, 17.18, and 18.21 used with permission from the photographer, Robert Cutter; all other photographs in Chapters 17 and 18 used with permission from the photographer, Claudine Laabs. Images of Valerie Gora in figures 17.15, 18.7, 18.20, and 18.27 used with permission from Valerie Gora. Figure 18.24 reprinted with permission by the artist, Josefine Frind.

Biodynamic Craniosacral Therapy, Volume Four is sponsored by the Society for the Study of Native Arts and Sciences, a nonprofit educational corporation whose goals are to develop an educational and cross-cultural perspective linking various scientific, social, and artistic fields; to nurture a holistic view of arts, sciences, humanities, and healing; and to publish and distribute literature on the relationship of mind, body, and nature.

North Atlantic Books' publications are available through most bookstores. For further information, visit our website at www.northatlanticbooks.com or call 800-733-3000.

MEDICAL DISCLAIMER: The following information is intended for general information purposes only. Individuals should always see their health care provider before administering any suggestions made in this book. Any application of the material set forth in the following pages is at the reader's discretion and is his or her sole responsibility.

New ISBN for Volume Four: 978-1-58394-373-1

Library of Congress Cataloging-in-Publication Data

Shea, Michael J., M.A.
  Biodynamic craniosacral therapy / by Michael J. Shea ; with contributions from Margaret Scott ... [et al.].
    p. ; cm.
  Includes bibliographical references and index.
  Summary: "A thorough description of the evolution of cranial osteopathic medicine into a new form available to many health care providers, this book presents a technique of touch therapy that is extremely gentle and subtle and gives practical exercises to be proficient in healing physical, spiritual, and emotional conditions"—Provided by publisher.
   ISBN-13: 978-1-55643-591-1
   ISBN-10: 1-55643-591-6
1. Craniosacral therapy. I. Society for the Study of Native Arts and Sciences. II. Title.
  [DNLM: 1. Complementary Therapies—methods. 2. Musculoskeletal Manipulations. 3. Mind-Body Relations (Metaphysics) 4. Sacrum. 5. Skull. WB 890 S539b 2007]
RZ399.C73S54 2007
615.8'2—dc22
                            2006031902

1 2 3 4 5 6 7 8 9 VERSA 16 15 14 13 12

This book is dedicated to His Holiness, the fourteenth Dalai Lama.

Whoever has great compassion can extinguish all obstructions caused by past actions and can fulfill all virtues; no principle cannot be understood, no path cannot be practiced, no knowledge not attained, no virtue not developed.

—Zen Master Torei

CONTENTS

SECTION III: PHOTOGRAPHIC TEXT-ATLAS OF BIODYNAMIC SKILLS

ILLUSTRATIONS

ACKNOWLEDGMENTS

I am very grateful to the numerous contributions from my team—family, students, editors. I acknowledge especially the calmness and courtesy of Emily Boyd at North Atlantic Books, who can answer every question without fail and give me every extension I ask for. Winn Kalmon, the copyeditor of this volume and all preceding volumes in this series, has brought a necessary precision and discriminating awareness to my writing. I am very grateful to have her hand, mind, and eyes on this and all my books.

This is a book of photography by Claudine Laabs (Figure A.1). The 142 photo illustrations in this book were taken over a twenty-year period. Claudine is one of South Florida's premier nature photographers. We first met when I was teaching yoga classes back in the mid-1970s and, since then, she has shared her love of the wildlife of South Florida with me, my wife Cathy, and many other people. Claudine has very graciously contributed the photograph of a bird called a skimmer (Figure A.2). It's really an amazing bird, flying along the shoreline with part of its beak in the sand as it gathers its food. It is a sight to behold when the ocean is calm. She likes to call it the slimming skimmer.

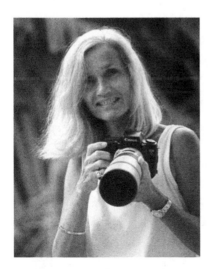

Figure A.1. Photographer Claudine Laabs

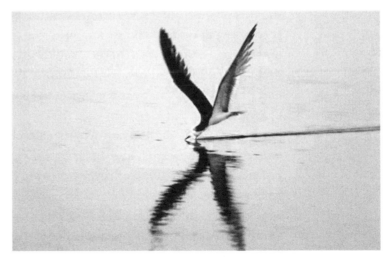

Figure A.2. Slimming skimmer

In addition, my friend Robert Cutter graciously contributed three photographs to this volume. Robert is an artist, acupuncturist, and biodynamic craniosacral therapist practicing in Santa Barbara, California. Thank you Robert.

Since it is the digital age, it was possible to touch up quite a few of the photographs, especially to eliminate the metal parts holding the skeleton together and edges and corners of the original photographs. To that end, Jeanie Burns did a remarkable job cleaning up almost half of the photographs, eliminating distracting elements in the background and making sure that the photographs that were originally taken with regular film were digitized properly. This turned out to be a significant amount of work with Volume Four. In addition, Jeanie created all the figures for Chapters 5 and 9.

I am very grateful as always to my family. My brother Brian, who is a sounding board for all that is biodynamic in this book and in life, is a true soul brother and has a magnificent pair of hands and equally bright mind. My sister Sheila, who contributed the first four chapters, has a powerful voice in the community of healers. Sheila was the person who helped launch my career by pointing me in the direction of my body and manual therapy. I am forever indebted to her for her generosity. I am gifted with her love and that of both my brothers Brian and Dan.

I simply could not have done this book without the brilliant help of Sara Dochterman. Sara has had her hand in all of my books but no more so than this one. From typing the whole manuscript, proofreading it (over and over), formatting it for submission, entering all the references in the bibliographic software, to reminding me to breathe when I was at my edge with the project, she has been completely present. She has been a secure anchor in my life during this project. Sara is a Licensed Clinical Social Worker in the state of Florida who very generously takes time out of her schedule to help me. She feeds me and I feed her meals whenever I can. She has even begun to work on Volume Five! I have included her contact information in the Resources section at the end of this book for anyone who would like clinical supervision or psychological counseling.

Once again I have received generous contributions from Friedrich Wolf, who drew the cover art, and Tim Shafer, who has reviewed numerous chapters, especially the Glossary, and always provides valuable insights and changes. Tim has been a teacher in training with me for almost ten years and I recognize him as a teacher of biodynamic craniosacral therapy. Congratulations, Tim. His contact information can also be found in the Resources section. Another amazing human being is Carol Agneessens. She has contributed to my other books and continues to contribute to my life with her honesty and integrity. She wrote Chapter 10 and continually dialogs with me about teaching the living embryo to our students. She is the best female teacher of this embryonic perspective in North America. She is a gift of loving kindness to all who encounter her. Her contact information can also be found in the Resources section.

I am also blessed to have two friends and biodynamic teachers in Europe, Catherine Vitte and Marcel Bryner. They understand the embryo and Primary Respiration at a profound level and their insight fills this book and inspires me to continue writing. I am also very grateful to all the help that Valerie Gora has provided in the formation of this book, especially in the last two photo shoots. Her hands and face appear in three photographs. Her contact information is also located in the Resources section. Valerie has been a teacher in training with me for almost ten years and she is now graduated as a full instructor of biodynamic craniosacral therapy. Congratulations, Valerie. She is an excellent teacher without a doubt. I also want to profoundly thank my office manager, Lisa Fay, who is a prayer in my life and keeps everything afloat as I disappear to write or travel and teach. Lisa's grace that she lives infuses this book.

As the reader will notice, the vast majority of photographs (ninety!) are of my hands on my wife Cathy. The photos span the twenty-one years of our marriage, starting just before we were married to the last photo shoot for this book in the summer of 2010. We always asked Claudine at the end of a photo shoot to take a picture of the two of us simply as a couple. I chose Figure A.3 from the last photo shoot as my favorite to include here. In addition, the viewer will note that all of the photos were taken with natural lighting. All the shoots were taken outdoors except for the very last one in the summer of 2010 and that one with only natural lighting.

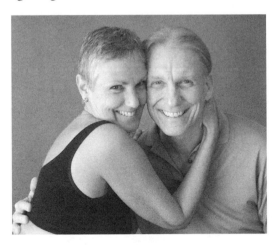

Figure A.3. Cathy and Michael Shea

Finally, I dedicate this book to Cathy and our twenty-one years of marriage. I spent so much time looking at the ninety photographs of her in this book that I kept learning to love my wife over and over again. I hope the viewer will appreciate the beauty that radiates from her in all of the photographs.

INTRODUCTION

This book is about the aesthetics of biodynamic practice. It is a photographic text-atlas of craniosacral therapy hand positions and descriptions of practicing biodynamically. The supporting text attempts to clarify the core biodynamic practices and perceptual processes as I teach them. I am also introducing a new metaphor regarding clinical biodynamic practice. It is the metaphor of *taking the pulse* of the client's fluid body much like an acupuncturist takes the meridian pulses of the client at the beginning and end of an acupuncture treatment. Consequently, I am using the term *pulse* and recommend that practitioners evaluate their client's fluid body in this way. Numerous chapters refer to taking different pulses all located within the fluid body. Some pulses are associated with traditional hand positions and some pulses refer more to different perceptual processes such as ignition or three-dimensional breathing of the fluid body occurring under the guidance of Primary Respiration. In this way, practitioners can further develop their clinical skills by determining if a change has been made in the client's fluid body at the end of a session.

This book is intended for all of my students past, present, and future. All of you have asked me for so many years to provide photographs and descriptions of all the hand positions that I teach in class. While this book in no way covers all the hand positions I teach, it covers a lot of ground, as the reader will see. I chose to show my own evolution and development of teaching craniosacral therapy over the past twenty-five years right up to the present. All form and styles of craniosacral therapy are valid. The issue is knowing when to apply it in a sequence of work, especially in biodynamic practice. I personally recommend doing mechanical, functional, or Mid Tide work in the middle of a biodynamic session as I teach it with Primary Respiration if it is even necessary. Many practitioners come to biodynamic practice by learning mechanical work first. Thus there are pictures of the traditional vault hold and the traditional CV4. There are also practitioners who only learn to work with the slow tide and thus I show the embryological seams taught in biodynamic practice.

I actually never thought there would be a Volume Four when I started writing a decade ago. Students always asked me how and where I find the time to write these books. It is quite simple. I like to create outlines for the lectures I give in class. I write the outline down on a flip chart in class, give the lecture, and then take notes or record the lecture. At that point, it either gets transcribed or dictated to my assistant and then I simply revise it five to ten times before I feel it is ready to hand out to students. I have hundreds of such essays and articles that I have written, and since the field of biodynamic craniosacral therapy is constantly changing and transforming, under the guidance of Primary Respiration and stillness, it seems as if the fountain of creativity and inspiration has no beginning and no end. And yes, there will be a Volume Five—work on it has already begun.

This book has three sections. Section I consists of four chapters written by my sister Sheila Shea. Like my wife Cathy, Sheila is a colon hydrotherapist. I have asked her to contribute these chapters because of the dire need I see in my clients and hear about from my students' clients regarding the rehabilitation of their fluid bodies. Inflammatory conditions and related disorders are epidemic in human bodies and thus the fluid body lacks ignition. Sometimes it is simply not enough to allow Primary Respiration to resuscitate the fluid body. The client, the practitioner, and many of us need help from the inside out and this can begin with simple dietary changes and basic information regarding how the gut becomes inflamed and can be the source of so many problems in the fluid body. I really enjoyed the revision process with my sister and the information is very important for the health and well-being of all human bodies.

Section II is about the art and aesthetics of applied biodynamic practice. I have attempted to minimize the theoretical component of this section and give as much practical information as possible. Chapter 5 has eight concept maps depicting the zones, which are boundaries of awareness in biodynamic practice. It is crucial that the practitioner periodically move some of his or her attention away from the physical contact and out the window to nature and back in the tempo of Primary Respiration. This theme is repeated throughout Section II. It is called a *cycle of attunement,* which is detailed in Chapter 6. A cycle of attunement is the basic unit of perceptual work and as such is a mindfulness practice in a biodynamic session. It simply involves periodically and consciously moving one's attention through the zones in present time.

During 2009 and 2010, I had the great privilege to be a member of the Massage Therapy Body of Knowledge task force. This task force was put together by the six leading organizations regulating massage therapy in the United States. The Body of Knowledge sets forth a set of basic competencies for the entire profession. Based on my learning curve during that time, I wrote Chapter 7, specifically for biodynamic practitioners. What I found in the neurological literature is the importance of understanding mirror neurons and applying that understanding to the therapeutic relationship. Mirror neurons are considered to be the biggest discovery since DNA in the science of the human body. Mirror neurons in the brain and heart are the foundation of empathetic and compassionate responses to the pain and suffering in people and thus our clients. Compassion is an innate part of human biology. I presented this research at the Massage Therapy Foundation Research Conference in Seattle, Washington in May 2010. What I said is that there is enough evidence to support the contention that massage therapy and, in the context of this book, biodynamic craniosacral therapy both can now be considered to be therapeutic models of empathy and compassion. This is discussed not only in Chapter 7, but Chapters 8 and 9 as well.

It is important to make distinctions between different levels of perception in biodynamic practice. Since it is an empathy- and compassion-based model, that means practically that the therapeutic relationship and healing in general depend much more on the conscious somatic awareness of the practitioner than on the client's innate health to manifest. Ignition is the subject of Chapter 9 and I have written extensively about it in my previous volumes. The more I practice with Primary Respiration, the more I see the distinction between combustion, ignition, and initiation. Combustion relates to the disturbances in the fluid body because of inflammatory processes and stress physiology. The energy of combustion needs to be transformed into ignition. Then there is ignition itself, which I define as a *transition state* (or states) between the phases of Primary Respiration as well as its constant interchange with stillness. Ignition is the reactor core, so to speak, of the therapeutic process discussed in Chapter 21. Finally, the whole issue of illness being an initiatory experience takes on a whole new light when it is considered as an ignition. All of life's transitions have the possibility to be ignitions. What gets ignited? The health that is preexisting in the body is allowed to manifest more potently. Health is none other than the expression of Primary Respiration in the fluid body. Chapter 9 is not only a synopsis of all that I have written about ignition, but is a clarification and a simplification for clinical practice.

Once again, Carol Agneessens has made a significant contribution to the field of biodynamic practice with her addition of Chapter 10 on holographic touch. Practitioners spend so much time attending to the fingers, palms, and ventral surface of the hands that it is easy to forget that in biodynamic practice, the hands need to be buoyant and transparent. One way to achieve that is to place attention on the dorsal or back surface of the hands and arms and body in general. I even do exercises in class in which the practitioner turns his or her back to the client and senses Primary Respiration from the client with the back of the practitioner's body. I then have the practitioner touch the client with the backs of his or her hands, even while he or she is sitting with back to the client. I recommend everyone try this experiment and do a session with the back of the hands and body. Carol, in elegant detail, points out the necessity for this type of palpatory skill in biodynamic practice and offers explorations to develop seeing, thinking, and knowing hands.

Both Volumes Two and Three have dedicated chapters to instructing the client on how to be with a biodynamic session. Chapter 11, on what I call horizon therapy, is another set of instructions to help guide the client in finding his or her body three dimensionally and forming a relationship with Primary Respiration. Biodynamic practice is not fix-it work; it is self-regulation and containment work. The scientific findings of interpersonal neurobiology are very clear that the practitioner and client are in a merged state and the priority is for the practitioner to maintain a significant degree of conscious somatic awareness during any session in order to differentiate from the client. To do so requires self-regulation skills on the part of the practitioner and the client. This builds resonance that allows the client the opportunity to synchronize with Primary Respiration and stillness in his or her own way. This is the same mechanism that the brains of mothers and babies use to grow and develop. This capacity never goes away. It is vitally important to teach the client how to form a personal relationship with Primary Respiration in order to integrate a session more thoroughly. In that way, biodynamic practice becomes a joint practice or a communion between two people.

Finally, I finish Section II with several fluid-body meditations. Breathing is the oldest function in the human body and the practitioner must be able to self-ignite periodically by synchronizing his or her secondary respiration with Primary Respiration. In addition, this allows the third ventricle to ignite. I recommend these practices be done not only during a session with a client, but as a meditation practice between sessions or while at home.

Section III is a photographic text-atlas of biodynamic skills, divided into seven chapters. I highly recommend the reader look over the beginning of Chapter 13 on how to view the photographs before viewing or using the hand positions described. Clinical practice is a practice of wholeness, of being able to sense one's whole body while the hands are in contact with the client. Since the photographs offer precision in terms of hand placement, it must be remembered that, at all times, the practitioner is using his or her whole body as if an extension of the hands, or rather the hands as an extension of the whole body. Furthermore, in biodynamic practice, the hands and arms of the practitioner are not just "tools of the trade," but rather form an umbilical connection with the client in such a way that the therapeutic relationship becomes a *circulatory system,* as was discussed in Volume Three.

Chapters 14 through 19 show hand positions, or what are called *windows,* for different areas of the body. A window is the surface vantage point that the hands have for viewing the whole of the client. Some of the photographs have extensive annotations and others have very minimal descriptions. Again, I would refer the reader back to Chapter 13 to be thoroughly familiar with the prerequisites for each hand position if it is not mentioned in a subsequent instruction. It simply does not make sense to keep repeating the same basic instructions over and over again for all the photographs, although I do periodically remind the reader in each chapter of these prerequisites. Chapter 20 is an easy reference guide with a very short description of each photograph. I designed the book this way so that the practitioner could have a ready reference in the treatment room and be able to choose a short description as a quick reminder or have the longer descriptions available for more detail. Finally, Chapter 21 reviews the biodynamic therapeutic processes related to the various windows of hand contact. In this way the practitioner will know what the priorities are in a session.

At the end of the book, I have created a glossary of biodynamic terminology. This glossary is not in alphabetical order, but rather is based on different categories of perception having to do with biodynamic process or fluidic perception, the bodily processes of shaping of the whole, and finally the relational processes of empathy and compassion. Not only is biodynamic practice a model of empathy and compassion, it is a deeply embodied process directly related to the phenomenology of the body. This means the immediate lived experience of the body and not necessarily anatomy and physiology. The term *lived experience* refers to a view that acknowledges the multidimensional aspects of our experiences, the context in which our experiences occur, and the meaning our experiences have in our lives. This includes our experience of space, time, our lived bodies, and our relationships. Our *lived bodies* allow us to perceive, interact with, and understand our world, and to make meaning of our experiences. Our bodily experiences, and the meaning they have in our lives, in turn shape our perceptions and future experiences. These are the roots of biodynamic practice and its orientation to three-dimensional fluidic lived experiences. I also wish to acknowledge Ann Weinstein, who contributed the definition of lived experience.

I am very pleased to present this Volume Four to you and I dedicate any merit that may come from the application of these skills and abilities for the relief of pain and suffering on this planet to my teacher, His Holiness the Dalai Lama. Every morning, when I meditate on his image, I make this dedication as I pray to him for guidance in my life and my writing. Now I give it to you with love.

Please note: Throughout the book gender references to the practitioner and client are different in most chapters—that is, the practitioner might be a "she" and the client a "he," or the practitioner a "he" and the client a "she." Some chapters refer to practitioners in the plural, and thus avoid the gender distinction altogether. Still other chapters use the cumbersome "he or she" or "his or her" to avoid any supposition of gender. Readers will get used to the variability, hopefully.

SECTION I

. . .

Repairing the Fluid Body

CHAPTER 1

Dealing with Poor Intestinal Health

by Sheila Shea

Originally, this chapter was presented as a paper in 2002 in Tucson, Arizona at a conference called Intestinal Health through Diet. My brother Michael asked me to publish it in this book as a way to inform craniosacral therapists about whole-body patterns and behaviors, especially the gut influencing the fluid body. The original paper has been thoroughly revised and updated. Many of the quotations of Elaine Gottschall here are email responses from her on a listserv called SCD-list@longisland.com, which is no longer in operation after her death. The reader can get a feel for Elaine Gottschall and her clarity of thinking in her correspondence referenced throughout. Other quotes of hers are from a website www.healingcrow.com and there are selected quotes from her book *Breaking the Vicious Cycle* (Gottschall, 2007). All quotes are reprinted with permission. Finally, I mention many medical conditions and biological terms in these first four chapters. I have done my best to create a glossary at the end of Chapter 4 for the reader who is unfamiliar with terminology I use or if my in-text definitions are insufficient.

The purpose here is to introduce the Specific Carbohydrate Diet (SCD) as a primary solution for inflammatory bowel disease, which is epidemic in our culture. In this exploration, I will also mention what conditions come under this umbrella, what causes the problems in the first place, what options we have to heal our intestines, and the details of the SCD. Overall, the idea is to keep an open mind, see the big picture, and find how things relate rather than how they are different, whether it is symptoms or diseases or parts of the gut and entire body.

What Does Intestinal Health through Diet Mean?

My intestinal health is my ability to digest, absorb, and eliminate optimally. The foods we consume on a daily basis affect our health intimately, and the biggest influence on our genes is the last meal we had. Our skin protects us from the outside world, but what protects our inside world? The gut is our inner skin. What that means to me is that everything people eat has the potential to help or hinder their intestinal health. Although many factors can influence intestinal health such as stress and emotions, the overall approach in these four chapters is intestinal health through diet.

I would also like to speak from personal experience as much as possible. This means not only speaking from my own personal life but also as a professional colon hydrotherapist for the past thirty-five years. In that time I have seen thousands of clients struggling with health through diet. What motivates me to make change, to focus on intestinal health through diet? I would say a few things motivate me. I was tired of being run by my addictions and eating disorders and not being in control of my own diet. I was motivated by a desire for freedom and choice when it came to food. I was pleasure motivated. I was tired of lack of quality of life from lifelong constipation. I was tired of the pain I would feel from gas, bloating, indigestion, and rectal bleeding. I politically did not want to support corporations that manufacture food that is deleterious to my health. So, freedom, pleasure, quality of life, and politics figured into my equation.

I searched all kinds of diets in order to discover what would be the right mix for me. I also began to practice some behavior modification in order to change food habits. It's easy to say food is something that we can control in our life, but it is not. I find it challenging to make dietary changes and so do my clients. It is important to acknowledge that emotions, thoughts, herbs, exercise, fetal development, breastfeeding (or lack thereof), genes, and other factors influence intestinal health. However, in these chapters, I am focusing on dietary aspects of intestinal health.

Hopefully, these chapters will provide tools to make better decisions about intestinal health. Hopefully, the reader will develop the discriminatory faculties such as mindfulness or simply begin paying conscious attention to eating and becoming more aware of gut sensations. Then by keeping one's self informed one can gradually develop the instinct about what is right for intestinal health and build the will and capacities or behaviors to practice them. This develops a critical neurological function and lifelong body awareness process called self-regulation. Self-regulation is a crucial element of everyone's bodily health; my brother Michael has written about it in his previous volumes. This sounds difficult but achieving intestinal health is a great victory and well worth it. It is another form of freedom!

What Are the Medical Options?

For gut problems surgery is a big one, with ostomies and resections that are no longer even viable options according to the latest research. You can have your intestines removed and a collecting bag installed (ostomy). Or you can have sections of your gut removed. You can spend a lifetime on medication such as Asacol and prednisone. Another big one is to ignore the problem. Ignoring only drives the problem deeper and one may develop related symptoms or diseases like migraines, chronic fatigue syndrome (CFS), allergies, rashes, weakened immunity, or hypothyroidism. However, these options do not target the *cause* or even risk factors; they merely remove, transfer, or reduce symptoms.

The solution that deals effectively with the cause of inflammatory bowel disease is *dietary*, especially the SCD. In Chapter 4, I will review other diet options and compare them briefly to SCD.

What Conditions May This Diet Help?

Inflammatory bowel diseases (IBDs) such as Crohn's disease, ulcerative and mucus colitis, cystic fibrosis, chronic diarrhea, diverticulitis, and celiac disease have a 75–80 percent recovery on the SCD. By the way, some terms are used interchangeably in bowel inflammation. IBD was formerly known as spastic colon and now accounts for more than half the visits to a gastroenterologist (Wise and Anderson, 2011). In addition, the terms *leaky gut* and *inappropriate permeability* have the same meaning as inflammation of the intestinal walls. The walls have been compromised in such a way that their integrity is damaged at a genetic level and substances ingested may now pass through the gut wall that were never intended to. Inflammation of the gut wall, leaky gut, and increased permeability are synonyms and one symptom of the inflammatory bowel disease and candida (yeast). I will address candida in Chapter 2.

Crohn's disease begins slowly, causing such symptoms as cramping abdominal pain, fever, fatigue, nausea, diarrhea, rectal bleeding, weight and/or appetite loss, and a chronic feeling of sickness. Crohn's disease tends to flare up and then subside, sometimes for months, before another episode occurs. Over time, the disease can cause abscesses and ulcers to form, which may then deeply erode the intestinal wall. In severe cases further complications, such as fistulas and anal fissures, can develop. Fistulas are abnormal passages between body organs that allow pus and fluids an avenue to drain in an attempt to eliminate them since the normal channels are not. In Crohn's disease, fistulas form between loops of intestine, intestine and skin, or intestine and bladder. Rarely, Crohn's disease-related inflammation and thickening of the small intestine are so severe that an intestinal obstruction occurs. Such an obstruction causes extreme abdominal pain with vomiting. Arthritis and skin lesions are systemic complications from Crohn's disease.

The SCD works well with irritable bowel syndrome (IBS). Gottschall made this comment about IBD and IBS: "As far as IBS being a completely different category from other IBD problems, I tend to think that all of them lie on a continuum … of everything in the human body as being connected in some way" (Gottschall, 2001). Begin to think of intestinal health in terms of the big or macro picture, in terms of relationships and continuums.

Oh et. al (1979) claimed that lactic acid formed from fermentation causes abnormal brain function and behavior that accompany so many intestinal disorders. Some intestinal disorders are associated with mental illness, ulcerative colitis with either schizophrenia or bipolar disorder, and chronic diarrhea with epilepsy. Some psychiatric, physical, and mental retardation symptoms show improvement. When the SCD is implemented, mental symptoms disappear first then intestinal.

Some immune conditions now show recovery with the SCD. Autism is one of the big crossover diseases. Originally thought to be a mental illness, autism is now considered an immune-mediated disorder. Recent research shows gut tissue samples that closely resemble Crohn's disease (Gottschall, 2007, p. 56). Clostridia, a pathogenic bacteria, and candida are found in the urine samples of people with autism. Recently, a number of children are in recovery from autism using the SCD (Gottschall, 2007, pp. 51–54). Other immune conditions responding to SCD are Epstein-Barr syndrome and/or chronic fatigue syndrome, fibromyalgia, lupus, and Behçet's syndrome.

The diet effectiveness has expanded to include seizures, allergies, candida, ankylosing spondylitis, arthritis, stomach ulcers from the *H. pylori* bacteria, high cholesterol, and hypothyroidism. Gottschall speculated that the SCD might be helpful in diabetes with restrictions to some single sugars and in multiple sclerosis because the diet is healthful and balanced. Many skin conditions respond to the diet such as dermatitis herpetiformis, psoriasis, eczema, and acne. Dermatitis herpetiformis is a symptom of celiac disease and appears in a symmetrical pattern on the skin preceded by excruciating itching.

I want to dwell more on celiac disease because we now have so much more information on this vastly underdiagnosed and serious condition. Celiac disease is an inflammatory bowel disease and an autoimmune condition in which the *intestinal brush border* (intestinal villi) has been flattened or blunted. Malabsorption, the inability to absorb vital nutrients, is a key result. Some of the symptoms might be diarrhea, constipation, rashes, gas, bloating, weight loss, mouth sores, migraines, depression, thyroid disease, diabetes, weight loss, short stature or inability to grow according to one's age, epilepsy, arthralgia (joint pain), anemia, and fatigue.

Dr. David Sanders and colleagues at the Gastroenterology and Liver Unit at the Royal Hallamshire Hospital in Sheffield, England assessed the association of celiac disease with IBS in patients fulfilling internationally designed criteria. "We now recognize typical, atypical, latent, and potential forms of celiac disease. At present, this disease is considerably underdiagnosed. The implications of missed diagnoses are the potential complications of osteoporosis, infertility, and an increased risk of malignant disease," according to the article in *Lancet* (Sanders, 2001, as referenced in McConnell, 2001). Gottschall referred to the book of her mentor, Dr. Haas, called *The Management of Celiac Disease* and a medical dictionary. Table 8 in Dr Haas's book lists all symptoms of celiac especially avitaminosis (inability to absorb vitamins) that accompany celiac disease. Also listed are sweating, edema, erythema, hives, photophobia, and stomatitis.

Stomatitis is inflammation of the mucous membrane of the mouth. The definition describes angular stomatitis as inflammation at the corners of the mouth usually superimposed over a wrinkled or fissured epithelium, stopping at the mucocutaneous junction and not involving the mucosa. Now we have more relationships with celiac—skin disease, avitaminosis, and stomatitis—that formerly might not be associated with celiac. How often do people get various chancres, sores, and cracks on their lips and not associate them with their gut health?

Robert Dahl, MD, spoke to a celiac group in Tucson where I live. He said in his talk that celiac disease may cause lesions and neuropathies in the cerebellum and peripheral nerves. Plus, "In untreated mothers there is an increased risk of low birth weight and intrauterine growth retardation (IUGR)." IUGR is a serious and significant indicator of long-term health. The placenta changes its genetic makeup and many diseases result from the maternal stress that causes IUGR. Recent research has suggested that 20 percent of all newborn babies have an inflammatory condition in their intestines (Savino et al., 2007; Rhoads et al., 2009; Savino et al., 2010). This is the most immediate complication from IUGR. In addition, one of my internet friends has a teenage daughter who was born with diabetes. She persuaded her GI doctor to test all his diabetic patients for celiac disease after she discovered that 5–7 percent of people with diabetes are prone to celiac disease.

Michael Toogood from the UK was originally diagnosed with Crohn's disease and ulcerative colitis only to find out later that he had celiac disease. He told a great story and gave outstanding links for further education on his website, which is no longer available. Here are a couple of quotes of his:

> If too many celiacs are diagnosed, we upset the food marketing industry, the beer industry, and the farming industry.
>
> I noticed that a lot of discipline would be needed to change the modern western diet of chemicals and stodge as radically as some of the dietary regimes asked. I back-pedaled on the idea of a radical diet, and carried on as the Hospital Dietician had advised.

Toogood expresses the difficulty many people have in changing their diet to save their life and intestinal health. He had diarrhea so bad that he could not even go for job interviews. Now I know some readers are thinking *But that's not my problem. I have constipation.* It is important to talk about one's intestinal condition. It is crucial to break the taboo of silence around one's intestinal health and condition.

What about babies and children? The SCD is helpful here too.

> Some of the most dramatic and fastest recoveries have occurred in babies and young children with severe constipation and among children who, along with intestinal problems, had serious behavior problems. [That sounds like my childhood!] These included autistic-type hypoactivity as well as hyperactivity, often accompanied by severe and prolonged night terrors.
>
> (Gottschall, 2007, pp. 1–2)

Hirschsprung's disease is a congenital disorder of the colon in which certain nerve cells, known as ganglion cells, are absent, causing chronic constipation. Hirschsprung's disease is suspected in a baby who has not passed meconium within forty-eight hours of delivery. When asked about Hirschsprung's disease in an infant, Gottschall responded on the listserv:

> I have had two babies reversed of this terrible disease with the infant formula at the back of the book [Gottschall, 2007]. Severe constipation also responds. My hypothesis is that what is called neonatal paralysis of the musculature that allows propulsion of the bowel movement (the medical community thinks you are born with it) is actually a change in the pH (acidity, alkalinity) of the environment surrounding the nerve-muscle activation. One of my students came to me many years after they had operated on her as a baby for this. She had by that time about twenty surgeries for draining fistulae of the abdomen. SCD reversed them.
>
> (Gottschall, email, 9/21/01, Re: Question OT Hirschsprung's Disease)

Consistency of stool is another indicator of celiac disease. Gottschall said to one of the listserv members, "Your baby does not have diarrhea if the stools are mushy but it sure is one of the pointers to celiac." I would say that if a baby has mushy stools, it may be an indicator of an inflamed intestine.

The *freezing* of the parasympathetic nervous system from early childhood trauma after birth goes hand in hand with many inflammatory bowel problems as well as chronic constipation (Scaer, 2001, 2005; Kirkengen, 2010). We know the muscles of the intestinal tract must contract and relax for peristalsis but they are dependent on the nerve stimuli in the gut and from the parasympathetic nervous system coming down from the brain stem. Childhood trauma and neglect thwart the body's ability to digest and eliminate properly. Everyday stress plays a major role in how effective peristalsis operates. Chronic stress as well as traumatic stress can shut down peristalsis via the activity of the autonomic nervous system, especially the parasympathetic nervous system. I do not have time to go into detail in the anatomy and neuorophysiology of the gut but the reader should take time to review it.

While Gottschall was alive, she shared her thoughts on an internet listserv called SCD-list@longisland.com as I mentioned before. She was very active in her email communications until two years before her death in 2005 at age 85. One member of that listserv on the SCD shared this story about his ulcerative colitis (UC). Sciatica, joint inflammation, and overweight were associated with his UC.

> I developed sciatica after developing UC. Since I have been on the SCD and over a long time, the sciatic pain and numbness have virtually disappeared. Somewhere recently, in some medical reference book, it mentioned that UC can also cause inflammation in a joint somewhere near the base of the spine. I am now thinking the sciatica may have been a symptom of the UC. Of course, I also went from about 185 pounds to about 150 pounds on the SCD, so that could be a factor, too.

Primary sclerosing cholangitis (PSC) is diagnosed in 70–80 percent of patients who are diagnosed with IBD. Cholangitis is an infection of the common bile duct, the tube that carries bile from the liver to the gall bladder and intestines. PSC is a chronic liver disease caused by progressive inflammation and scarring of the bile ducts of the liver. The inflammation impedes the flow of bile to the gut, which can ultimately lead to liver cirrhosis, liver failure, and liver cancer. Doctors believe it is caused by an overactive immune system. A few cases are recovering on the SCD.

Malabsorption is a result of bowel inflammation and can be reversed by the SCD. Gottschall wrote on the listserv that "overgrowth of microbes on the intestinal wall cause inflammation and inability to absorb and transport essential nutrients and thus leads to vitamin and mineral deficiencies." She continued:

> It's my joke about the ankle bone being connected to the neck bone! Anyone lucky enough to have found Dr. Haas's book, *The Management of Celiac Disease* [Haas and Haas, 1951], would find that the thyroid gland is one of the first organs of the body to suffer the effects of malabsorption and/or lack of sufficient essential nutrients. It is hoped that as the SCD reverses the malabsorption, the thyroid will come back. Have it checked periodically because it is very common to find that the thyroid medication must be decreased as one begins to absorb nutrition and recover.
> (Gottschall, email, 10/21/01, Re: Thyroid Disease and UC)

The association of thyroid deficiency with intestinal malabsorption implies that other endocrine imbalances might result from inflammatory bowel disease. Most people with IBD at some point can become deficient in a whole array of nutrients due to the malabsorption resulting in symptoms such as spasms, cramps, edema, and many more. Magnesium deficiency can cause the colon muscles to contract strongly or spasm, potassium aids peristalsis, and a magnesium deficiency causes decreased potassium levels. Spasms and decreased peristalsis are a part of many inflammatory bowel diseases.

Malabsorption creates vitamin and mineral deficiencies. No cellular actions can be performed without cofactors that are in vitamins and minerals, many of which are manufactured in a normal healthy intestine. The gut and the liver are often at the bottom of eye problems and some hearing challenges. Many eye problems, like sensitivity to light, clear up on the SCD.

Many symptoms are addressed with the SCD, including, gas, bloating, abdominal pain, indigestion, alternating constipation and diarrhea, constipation alone, intestinal bleeding, weight loss, and fever. One definition of constipation is a decrease in the frequency of passage of formed stools and by stools that are hard and difficult to pass (McMillan, 2004). Constipation and diarrhea respond to the diet, as they are two extreme symptoms that likely have a common cause. Those with celiac disease and even those with ulcerative colitis and chronic diarrhea usually go through periods of constipation as well.

It's important to note that gut tissue is composed of 60–70 percent immune tissue. Therefore, what people are doing to their gut they are also doing to their immune system. If people are destroying their gut through diet, they are also destroying their immune system. That is why many immune conditions respond to the SCD. It helps to rebuild the gut wall. Also, many of the conditions that respond to the SCD are *inflammatory* conditions of the intestines or other parts of the body. Sites of inflammation in the body can trigger symptoms anywhere in the body and if the source is the gut then the SCD will not only heal the gut but also relieve systemic aches and pains caused by gut inflammation. Many conditions piggyback in a person with IBD such as sciatica, skin conditions, diabetes, cholangitis, and so forth.

_____

Reprinted with permission from Sheila Shea. Quotes by Elaine Gottschall reprinted with permission.

CHAPTER 2

The Problem Defined

by Sheila Shea

What Causes Poor Intestinal Health?

In Chapter 1, I mentioned many conditions that are far short of normal intestinal health and which respond to the SCD. What might cause these conditions to occur? That is what I want to deal with in this chapter. The basic theory underlying the SCD is that disease-producing bacteria and fungus gain control in the intestines when their natural balance has been disrupted. Some of the factors that disrupt balance in the gut are:

- Complex carbohydrate indigestion
- Overeating, food addictions, and eating disorders
- Antibiotics
- Parasites, harmful bacteria, or yeast from food or water
- Toxic chemicals in food or water
- Immune suppression from disease, malnutrition, or stress
- Aspirin, NSAIDs, vaccines
- Antacids

Another theory is that the dramatic increase in irritable bowel disease that has taken place in the last fifty years parallels the increasing use of antibiotics in human and veterinary medicine (and then we eat the meat from these animals). Antibiotics can promote the proliferation of toxic bacteria like salmonella and can make them more invasive. They can also cause mutation of bacteria and bacterial resistance. Hardly a month goes by without another bacterial outbreak in the food chain in this country. Even yesterday as I was finishing writing this chapter I read that thirty million pounds of frozen turkey meat was being recalled because of a salmonella outbreak that hospitalized a number of people.

One person reported on the listserv that he felt his problem is due to leaky gut syndrome triggered by taking large amounts of aspirin for leg and knee pain caused by running: "My IBS began about six months after I began the aspirin regimen." Epidemiological studies have implicated measles vaccine as a possible cause of increased risk of IBD. Some research has linked autism and IBD that has followed measles/mumps/rubella vaccinations. This statement is controversial in the literature and should be recognized as such. I tell parents to gather as much information as they can about vaccinations and then make an informed decision.

New unnatural substances have been introduced into our gastrointestinal tracts. These include fluoridated and chlorinated water, the residue of dental fillings containing mercury, traces of other materials used in dental work, toothpaste residues in the intestinal mucosa containing aluminum, silicon, and titanium, antacids containing aluminum, food additives, and synthetic food ingredients. Corn syrup, Olestra, and MSG fit into the additive category. Over time these substances can be highly destructive to the gut. Many of these substances also cause an overgrowth of bacteria in the mouth that has been linked to heart disease.

Adrenal hormones such as epinephrine can shut down digestion. Many people today experience chronic stress in their life and do not respond well to it. The adrenals become activated under stress and draw blood from the core viscera including the gut and redirect the blood flow to the extremities, the musculoskeletal system. It's the old fight-or-flight reaction that drains core energy from the gut and preps our muscles and nerves to respond to a threat. When this happens, our intestines are abandoned for our arms and legs. Digestion, absorption, and elimination are severely compromised with chronic stress until hormonal balance and blood flow to the core are restored. Even then there may be long-term damage to the gut because it is rare for people under stress to eat a healthful diet. Gottschall wrote on the listserv in 2000:

> Second lesson in endocrinology: Under stress, the adrenals produce adrenaline, epinephrine, which shunts blood with nutrients and oxygen away from intestine to arms and legs for fight and flight. That gives ample opportunity for anaerobic microbes to gain control in the gut. So prolonged stress could amplify the causes of IBD or exacerbate the conditions.
>
> (Gottschall, email, 9/19/00, Re: Stress and its effects)

People who eat at fast-food restaurants regularly and who eat too much sugar may increase their risk of Crohn's disease and ulcerative colitis, according to Persson, Ahlbom, and Hellers (1992). The baseline in the research was two fast-food meals per week and a total of fifty-five grams of sugar per day. Many other factors can cause bowel inflammation, leaky gut, or inappropriate permeability. According to Gottschall, complex carbohydrates are the major culprit in IBD. Recent European research has verified Gottschall's findings (Bentz et al., 2011; Demetrius, Coy, and Tuszynski, 2010; Xu et al., 2009), demonstrating that a gene in complex carbohydrates feeds certain kinds of cancer tumors. This gene can also cause metastes or spreading of the cancer tumors to occur. Such tumors can shrink from the elimination of complex carbohydrates in one's diet. However, it is important to note how other factors in one's life might be influential crosscurrents. Being proactive with one's health and practicing the SCD can always help.

Gottschall presented her theory of causation:

I feel that the bacteria and other microorganisms at the bottom of this are mutations of normal intestinal bacteria. We have published reports of any number of normal bacteria such as Escherichia coli developing mutations, adhering tenaciously and abnormally to the gut wall and producing toxins because of taking antibiotics or other medications. I think one way they can mutate is a result of having the acidity of the colon increase by the fermentation acids created by bacteria attacking unabsorbed illegal carbohydrates. This has been shown to happen in grain-fed cattle.

(Gottschall, email, 10/3/01, www.healingcrow.com, Re: Cheese and Mycobacterium Paratuberculosis)

Try to find time to read some of the information on *Giardia* and Enteroameba histolytica. I think it is far more important than worrying about yeast. They are all in this together but I still think the protozoan parasites and mutated bacteria are at the bottom of most of these UC cases and perhaps some of the Crohn's. But whatever, stay on SCD because the carbohydrates are certainly implicated in supporting the growth of all three: protozoan parasites like *Giardia* and *Amoeba* as well as the anaerobic bacteria and yeast.

(Gottschall, email, 5/27/00, Re: Vitamins/I need ideas/Linda)

Clostridium and *Klebsiella* are two bacteria that may also be implicated in IBD and other conditions. *Clostridium dificile* is a bacterium that causes serious bowel problems such as ulcerative and pseudomembraneous colitis. It belongs to a family of bacteria that are spore formers, which means they can hibernate in a shell-like case if things like nutrition are not to their liking. Not a normal inhabitant of the gut, this bacterium must mutate from another type. It is a result of taking antibiotics to which this bacterium becomes resistant. Once a bacterium mutates and becomes antibiotic resistant, it usually develops survival characteristics such as claw-like appendages that hook onto the gut wall and are not removed by the normal muscle movement of peristalsis. They also produce toxins and waste products that not only inflame the bowel wall but also enter the cardiovascular system and cause all kinds of metabolic and physiological problems.

An article on the SCD website Healing Crow, by Seth Barrows, called "The Great Yogurt Conspiracy" (Barrows, 2001) postulates that ankylosing spondylosis and increased intestinal permeability are possibly caused by a "bad" bacteria, *Klebsiella*, the growth of which is encouraged by inulin/fructooligosaccharides (FOS). I will discuss FOS in the next chapter.

One listserv member wrote Gottschall: "I was under the impression that colitic arthritis is not the same thing as rheumatoid arthritis (although I was tested and have antibodies for RA also). I'm confused as to whether or not I should be treating this disease as colitis or as arthritis."

Gottschall responded on the listserv:

Every so often, we have to get back to perspectives of medical diagnosis. It is based on either micro thinking or macro thinking. Since both colitis and Rheumatoid Arthritis are looked upon as a response of the immune system against the self—or autoimmune—many researchers believe that although the symptoms appear in different locations, it is still the immune cells attempting to destroy overgrowth of intestinal bacteria and in so doing activate the immune system to self-destruct. You should be treating the disease according to what it is: an overgrowth in intestinal bacteria that has become an autoimmune disease. Remedy: get rid of the overgrowth.

(Gottschall, email, 10/15/01, Re: Colitic Arthritis)

One listserv member asked Gottschall how she could go from feeling so fatigued on one diet, and then switch to the SCD and feel a new energy. The response on the listserv revealed new research on human digestion versus rumen digestion. Another bacterium was implicated in this plot. Gottschall explained that fatigue converts to more energy when the person reverts to human digestion rather than a rumen type of digestion.

If we do not absorb glucose molecules from starch, disaccharides, or even monosaccharides from our absorptive small intestine, they go down to the microbial world of the colon. Glucose molecules containing the greatest amount of energy are converted to volatile fatty acids by bacteria or yeast in the lower part of the ileum and colon. This bacterial fermentation process is inefficient for giving you energy from calories of food.

Once you change the digestive process by starving the critters and absorbing legal sugars more efficiently, you will then be getting human digestion working correctly. Your cells will get thirty-eight molecules of Adenosine-5'-Triphosphate (ATP) from one molecule of glucose. That is the point when so many on SCD begin feeling so very energetic, unlike anything they have felt for a long time.

(Gottschall, email, 7/5/01, Re: Easing Initial Fatigue)

Gottschall hypothesized that chronic fatigue syndrome and fibromyalgia could result from the cellular and thus energy deprivation from fermentation digestion. I will discuss sugars at length in the next chapter.

A subclass of people with intestinal disorders have diarrhea and are overweight. Sixty-seven percent of Americans are now overweight. Obesity has now been definitively linked to prenatal stress and poor prenatal nutrition. Maternal stress greatly compromises the placenta and causes it to become inflamed. As mentioned in Chapter 1 this is called intrauterine growth restriction (IUGR). This inflammation is then passed through to the fetus and not just to the gut of the fetus (Wadhwa, 2005; Wadhwa et al., 2002). According to Gottschall, the fatty acids being fermented from the undigested, unabsorbed sugars and starches are turning into volatile fatty acid such as lactic, acetic, and butyric (small molecules but are fat soluble). They are high in calories like alcohol and can get through the intestinal colonic membrane quite easily. They can put fat on some people. It is like eating a gram of starch that is 4 kilocalories and after fermentation turns into a gram of fat that contains 9 kilocalories.

What exactly is rumen digestion? Cows have a rumen, the first stomach of two that are interconnected. In fact, all herbivores have a rumen. All the starch and sugar is broken down in the rumen by fermentation and the cow absorbs the fatty acids into its bloodstream. Then the food returns to its esophagus (chewing its cud) and travels beyond the rumen to its second stomach where digestion proceeds much like ours.

What is happening in human bowel problems is that we as omnivores are not supposed to have much bacterial digestion until the first part of the large intestine, the ascending colon. Because many people eat low-fat, high-carbohydrate or high-carbohydrate diets, we have overwhelmed the small intestine's ability to break down and absorb all that starch. Therefore, the starch goes down to the colon and becomes food for normal and pathogenic bacteria.

In Cornell University research (Diez-Gonzalez et al., 1998), it was found that if cattle are fed a high-grain (high-starch) diet the same kind of bacterial attack occurs on the oversupply of starch reaching the lower gut. As fermentation occurs, the acidity increases from the formation of organic short-chain fatty acids. As the acidity increases, the pH of the gut and body become unbalanced. This is called acidosis. It changes the characteristics of normal nonpathologic *E. coli* bacteria found in the gut and they become a threat. In other words, feeding beef and dairy cattle a high-grain diet instead of hay can change a *harmless* bacterium into a *harmful* one turning on some genes and turning off others. This is called epigenesis and it is a hot topic in science right now (Meaney, 2010).

Since the early 1980s, medical research has shown that some forms of ulcerative colitis appear to be caused by a commonly found intestinal bacterium, *Escherichia coli (E. coli)*, which, as a result of a change in its characteristics (a mutation), has developed the ability to produce acute sicknesses and even death. Although there are numerous reasons as to why harmless forms of bacteria might change their characteristics through genetic mutation, the question could be asked: Is the fermentation of undigested, unabsorbed starch by intestinal bacteria in the human colon causing an acidic environment which could cause harmless bacteria to change to harmful forms?

Humans are not supposed to have a rumen where bacteria digest the indigestible components of a diet like cellulose in herbivores like cows. However, because *we are not eating a diet that is compatible with our genetic makeup,* we have substituted the cecum of the large intestine for a rumen. As a result, the ileocecal valve in the cecum at the entrance to the large intestine, the appendix, and the ascending colon may become infected with this overgrowth of mutated normal bacteria. The ascending colon is attached to the ileum of the small intestine and that is where the classic cases of Crohn's disease start. That is also the site of vitamin B_{12} absorption. Recent research has indicated that there are three basic enterotypes regarding normal intestinal bacteria (Arumugam et al., 2011). In other words, the world's human population seems to have three different types of gut based on each one having a different mixture of healthful bacteria. The implications of this research are not known yet but it would be easy to speculate that diet plays a critical role in one's enterotype.

Gottschall commented: "The appendix has been studied for years by a small group of investigators who believe it is one of the most important immune organs in the body, not a vestigial nothing to be pulled out with the tonsils and adenoids! The appendix is connected to the ileocecal junction where Crohn's begins in most cases." I think that some cases of appendicitis are actually the beginning of some form of IBD for that person. In simple terms, cattle and humans are being fed a high-grain, starchy diet rather than completely sprouted grains or grasses. The cattle and human diets are part of a bigger picture, the grain economy. That is another story for another time but the documentary film *King Corn* will open the reader's eyes to the corporate grain economy.

The *Journal of Dairy Science* ran an article by New York state researcher James Nocek (1997) that also concurs with the Cornell research cited above. The article begins: "Top producing herds are walking, and sometimes limping, the fine line between profitable high milk yield and poor health because of subclinical acidosis." Acidosis from feeding too much grain shocks the cow's system, increasing blood pressure and destroying blood vessels in the feet, leading to laminitis. Nothing you can sprinkle over the cow or her feed will make it better. Nocek calls it "a permanent breakdown."

Candida

Some people ask questions about candida and the SCD, and others are concerned about bacteria and the diet. One new area of research, on what is called *biofilm,* has helped us to understand the relationship between the two types of dietary relationships. Gottschall responded to a listserv member question:

> Your questions about candidiasis, honey, and fruit are well taken. The great gurus out there have maintained that those sugars are bad and grains are OK. So, people are confused. I believe that if a person has a yeast infection in the mouth like thrush, they should eliminate the honey. But this stuff about fruit does not make scientific sense.
>
> (Gottschall, email, 9/4/01, Re: Candida)

I have consistently and constantly made the point that one always has an overgrowth of yeast (candida) with an overgrowth of bacteria and they live cozily together in a biofilm where they help each other out. If the yeast overgrows, so do bacteria. They live symbiotically in a biofilm on the gut surface protected from antibiotics and other medications by the biofilm. Dr. William Costerton has done extensive work on the biofilm (Costerton, 2007). The research on biofilm also shows the basis of how plaque is formed on teeth. It is the structural foundation for the house of unhealthful bacteria and yeast in the mouth and gut.

What's the Relation of Bowel Inflammation and Leaky Gut?

This is a *continuum* issue. The miracle of digestion is that when our GI system cannot break down sugars and starches with healthful bacteria and biochemistry, pathogenic bacteria and fungi will. But their by-products irritate and inflame the gut walls. I see excess permeability, leaky gut, and inflammation as different names or phases of the same condition. The results of this chain of events injure the gut wall and seep into our bloodstream causing symptoms and diseases that appear unrelated to the gut. Remember, it is a continuum. The intestinal epithelium is permeable in order for nutrition to reach the whole body. Normal substances from molecules to big fat cells move back and forth across this vast border.

Overpermeability opens up this vast border even more to larger unhealthier molecules. Unnatural substances that were never designed to enter the bloodstream can take a long journey through the body and take up housekeeping in such places as the liver, the first organ through which they pass, as well as in the brain, muscles, bones, and other organs. At the other end of the continuum, the gut may appear to act like the Great Wall of China. The blunting of the microvilli in celiac disease and the fibrosing of tissue in Crohn's disease can prevent movement and absorption in some areas of the gut. Neither the good nor the bad get in.

What Is the Vicious Cycle?

The presence of undigested carbohydrates in the small intestine encourages bacteria and yeast from the colon to take up residence in the small intestine and continue to multiply. Bacterial by-products in the small intestines destroy enzymes secreted by the microvilli on the intestinal cell surface so that digestion and absorption are nearly impossible and more fermentation occurs. At this point, mucus-producing cells in the small intestines, called *goblet cells,* kick in more strongly than normal. Their mucus secretions protect the intestinal wall against microbial toxins and undigested carbohydrates. The mucus coating prevents sugars and starches needing digestion from reaching the absorptive and enzyme cells. Fermentation and damage escalate and normal absorption of B_{12} is disturbed. Goblet cells may be disabled as irritation to the gut wall progresses. When this happens, the pathway is open for ulcerative colitis and the whole cascade of similar conditions that I have been talking about.

This is a double bind. Now, the enzymes in the microvilli cannot reach the food and the microvilli are injured and cannot secrete enzymes. So, fermentation, gut wall injury, and malabsorption become more severe. And the intestinal disorder is prolonged. This is the vicious cycle. The research by Dr. S. V. Haas and Gottschall advocate the SCD in altering the microbial growth both qualitatively and quantitatively. The SCD is intended to break this vicious cycle of gut destruction.

Reprinted with permission from Sheila Shea. Quotes by Elaine Gottschall reprinted with permission.

CHAPTER 3

The Solution Defined

by Sheila Shea

Two solutions are available for the problem conditions described in the preceding chapters. Gottschall said that the IBDs are an overgrowth of intestinal bacteria generating an autoimmune disorder. Her remedy is to treat the overgrowth. Eating in a way that decreases fermentation will rid the gut of changed, perhaps mutated, bacteria and let them return to their normal non-pathological form. The second solution is that in some cases detoxification will be necessary with the use of colonic irrigations. I have seen this help repeatedly in my thirty-plus years of being a colon hydrotherapist.

The SCD is designed to restore normal gut flora and therefore allow human digestion to occur. Quoting from Gottschall's book:

> The purpose of the SCD is to deprive the microbial world of the intestine of the food it needs to overpopulate. By using a diet which contains predominantly predigested carbohydrates, the individual with an intestinal problem can be maximally nourished without overstimulation of the intestinal microbial population.
>
> (Gottschall, 2007, p. 10)

The diet offers an 80 percent recovery rate for those who follow it. Gottschall formulated the diet based on personal experience with her daughter, who at age eight had advanced and debilitating ulcerative colitis. Faced with the imminent prospect of surgery to remove her daughter's colon and a lifetime of prescription medication, Gottschall took her daughter to many different specialists seeking a remedy.

It wasn't until she saw Dr. Sidney Valentine Haas that she found help. His approach went back to an early naturopathic tradition that recognized "pathogenic fermentation" as the root cause of gastrointestinal ailments. He informed her of the diet called the SCD to get at the root cause. The results were slow but remarkable. Her daughter's total recovery inspired Gottschall to spread the word of the SCD to others. She decided to enroll in graduate school to further research the diet. The publication of her book *Breaking the Vicious Cycle* (2007) has helped to inform millions of people about the diet.

Defining Specific Carbohydrates

Carbohydrates are a class of sugars and starches. Gottschall defines and describes three types of carbohydrates and how they affect the gut wall. The three sugars and starches are called monosaccharides, disaccharides, and polysaccharides. The disaccharides and polysaccharides are also known as complex carbohydrates or complex sugars. Those terms can be used interchangeably.

First are single sugars called *monosaccharides*. The bloodstream absorbs glucose, fructose, and galactose directly without needing further breakdown or digestion. Honey, fruits, and some vegetables contain glucose and fructose. Homemade yogurt contains galactose. All are safe and acceptable sugars for the gut. Monosaccharides are considered predigested carbohydrates.

Second are double sugars or *disaccharides*. The double sugars require splitting by intestinal cell enzymes. Two disaccharides most well known are lactose and sucrose from milk and refined sugar. The other two, maltose and isomaltose, result from the breakdown of starches by enzymes of the saliva and pancreas. Enzymes at the tips of small intestinal microvilli break down all four of these disaccharides into single sugars.

Third are the multiple sugars, *polysaccharides* or starches that are of two types: amylose and amylopectin. Potatoes, yams, and grains are polysaccharides. The derivatives of grain, such as pasta, bagels, cereals, popcorn, and bread are on this list. The intestinal enzymes required for digesting polysaccharides are in the shortest supply, even in a healthy gut. Starches that contain more amylose that amylopectin starch are simpler to digest because the glucose units that make them up are arranged in a linear fashion and are readily exposed to digestive enzymes from saliva and the pancreas.

By comparison, amylopectin molecules contain glucose units that form branches. The interior branches appear less exposed than the exterior branches. Therefore, it is possible that pancreatic digestive enzymes cannot reach the interior links and that parts of the amylopectin starch molecules escape digestion, remain in the intestines, and increase microbial fermentation. The amount of amylopectin starch is very high in grain; some corn contains only amylopectin. Rice and sweet potatoes are other examples.

Remember, digestion splits every one of the sugar glucose molecules from each other and only then can the glucose pass through the intestinal-wall villi and be picked up by the capillaries of the bloodstream to give the body caloric energy within each individual cell. The final step in the digestion of starch (after the pancreas and saliva have separated attached groups of glucose sugars) is to break down the remaining disaccharides that must be processed by the enzymes of the intestinal cells.

In most sick people and especially in people with IBD, the enzymes are very low or absent and therefore primarily the isomaltose, but also lactose, sucrose, and maltose cannot be broken from one two-sugar molecule to two one-sugar molecules. They therefore go down to the lower part of the gut and are attacked by bacterial and fungal microorganisms. The isomaltose is even hard for healthy people to split and, therefore, as people increase their ingestion of starch, it is most probable that most of the isomaltose is undigested and used as food by bacteria and yeast. In some cases, the proteins of certain plants may prevent the starch from being completely split.

The SCD requires eating foods that contain monosaccharides and proteins and fats. The result is a diet that supplies the body with healthful food and starves the pathogenic microbial flora. The SCD also encourages the use of fermented foods, especially homemade yogurt, and probiotics. Probiotics are the prepackaged healthful bacteria found in many grocery stores now and not just health food stores. Yogurt has traditionally been a source of healthful bacteria as well as many other types of fermented foods such as sauerkraut. The consumption of fermented foods and probiotics replaces the starving microflora with beneficial bacteria. Gottschall believed only in acidophilus as a probiotic. However, her successor Campbell-McBride, in her book *Gut and Psychology Syndrome* (2004), suggested a wide variety of flora should be taken. I recommend finding what works best for the individual as indicated by formed floating stool and a decrease in intestinal discomfort. One should try several brands that have different combinations until one's gut clicks with the right one.

The living culture in yogurt is good to restore the flora if one is not allergic to dairy products. In yogurt, lactose, a complex sugar, is fermented into galactose, a single sugar, and is thereby absorbed directly into the bloodstream. Gottschall said on the listserv:

> As for probiotics, Dr. S. V. Haas used them. Lactobacillus acidophilus has been shown through over one hundred years of research to be helpful. Also its cousin, Lactobacillus bulgaricus, is much the same as the other and in our yogurt is playing many parts: first, digesting the lactose and by the lowered pH making the milk protein, casein, more digestible, and

second, introducing a beneficial bacteria into the gut. Many people say that bulgaricus is only a transient bacterium and does not take up residence. I did many months of work on these two cousins and I do not think that is accurate. It depends on the gut environment as to which take up residence and squeeze out room the bad guys are taking up.

(Gottschall, email, 6/7/01, Re: Diets)

Given enough time, the SCD changes the nature of the microbial flora and gives the body the nutrients and microfloral environment needed to heal. If the intestines cannot absorb monosaccharides, then these too will lead to a microbial overgrowth. Candida and diabetes might be examples of this. In this case, a restricted low-carbohydrate diet would be needed.

Foods On and Off the Diet

The SCD indicates which sugars can be safely eaten and which ones cannot. The SCD allows the single-sugar or monosaccharide foods—fruits, vegetables, certain nuts, honey, and homemade yogurt. The volume eaten of these foods determines whether one's diet is high or low in carbohydrates. With candida or diabetes, one's volume intake of these single sugars might be low initially.

Some people use the terms *simple* and *single* sugars to mean the same thing. "Simple" in SCD vernacular implies complex sugars, such as white sugar, flour, and milk, that are more complex to digest. A single sugar is a single sugar molecule that is simple to digest because it passes right into the blood stream. Single sugars are fruits, vegetables, honey, and homemade yogurt.

ALLOWED FOODS IN THE SCD

Fruits	Most fruits except plantains
Sugars	Honey
Vegetables	Most vegetables, fresh or frozen, and raw or cooked
Legumes	Navy beans, lentils, peas, split peas, peanuts in a shell, natural peanut butter, lima beans, and string beans
Meats	Unprocessed meats, such as beef, pork, chicken, turkey, quail, ostrich, fish, shellfish, lamb, venison, and rabbit
Dairy	Natural cheeses cured and aged properly, such as cheddar, colby, swiss, havarti, dry curd cottage cheese (Gottschall 2007, p. 178); homemade yogurt fermented a minimum of 24 hours; eggs
Nuts	Almonds, Brazil nuts, walnuts, pecans, chestnuts, filberts, unroasted cashews, raw pistachios

Alcohol	On rare occasions a small amount of dry wine, gin, scotch whiskey, bourbon, and vodka
Miscellaneous	Olive oil, coconut oil, soybean oil, corn oil, weak tea, weak coffee, unflavored gelatin, mustard, vinegar, saccharin, and juices with no additives

DISALLOWED FOODS

Sugars	White sugar, molasses, sucrose, high-fructose corn syrup, fructose, any processed sugar, barley malt, rice syrup, maltodextrin
Vegetables	All canned vegetables; potatoes, sweet potatoes, yams, yucca, kudzu, seaweed, carrageenan, agar
Grains	All grains and flour products such as corn, wheat, wheat germ and bran, barley, oats and oat bran, rye, rice, buckwheat, amaranth, quinoa, spelt
Legumes	Fava beans, chickpeas (garbanzos), soybeans, mung beans, starchy sprouts
Meats	Canned, cured, and most processed meats. (Read label to ensure processed meat doesn't contain any harmful additive such as corn, corn products, starch, sugar, whey, nonfat dry milk, soy.)
Dairy	Whole, skim, 1 percent, 2 percent, chocolate milk, ricotta, mozzarella, cottage cheese, cream cheese, feta, processed cheeses and cheese spreads, commercial yogurt, heavy cream, buttermilk, and sour cream
Miscellaneous	Canola oil, commercial mayonnaise (additives), cocoa, chocolate, carob, whey powder, margarine, commercial ketchup, baking powder, mixed nuts, maltodextrin, and FOS (fructooligosaccharides) products

The SCD is *specific for certain carbohydrates*, which ones are included and which ones excluded. Allowed are single sugars such as fruits, vegetables, honey, and homemade yogurt. Not allowed are complex sugars such as starchy roots, grain and flour products, the legumes soy and chickpeas, white sugar, flour, and milk. Chocolate is not allowed because it has a predominance of complex sugars before sugar and milk are added.

Gottschall split hairs when it comes to sugars and once you get beyond a single molecule of a sugar, the more complex molecules or bonds, strands, and branchings of sugars do need splitting down to the single level if they are going to be food rather than gut bacteria and fungi. If single sugars are not being digested for any reason, including overeating, they too will be fodder for the microbial world of the terminal ileum and colon. In addition, the more complex sugars one eats the more they go direct to the liver for storage as fat. This leads to metabolic syndrome and insulin resistance at a cellular level.

Is insoluble cellulose in fruits and vegetables food for bad bacteria? Dr. Costerton, of University of Southern California and biofilm discoverer (Costerton, 2007; Costerton et al., 1995), plus other resources I have reviewed, say that some bacteria can break the cellulose and lignin of nonsoluble fiber and thrive on them. That's why at the beginning of the diet, Gottschall asked that fruits and vegetables have their skins removed and be cooked.

Cooking softens the rigid cell walls. Only when they are softened is there a chance that the vitamins, minerals, and sugars in foods can be "milked out" and absorbed into the bloodstream. Raw fruits and vegetables will pass through the 23 feet of small intestine without the small intestine being able to extract the sugars. The sugars will go down to the lower small intestine and colon and create too much carbohydrate for the bacteria there.

Raw fruit may be eaten if diarrhea and cramping are no longer experienced. That is because healing has taken place and normal movement through the gut has replaced hypermotility. Thus, the small intestine has the normal time to work on the raw fruit. Besides, you have already reduced or changed some of the culprit bacteria (anaerobes which thrive on carbohydrates) and even if some fruit sugars do get down there, you will not have the same reaction you had when you first went on the diet with overpopulation of culprits as well as a hypermotile gut.

Lactose intolerance is a lack of the enzymes necessary to digest lactose. Some individuals are unable to break lactose down into monosaccharides. Lactose, a disaccharide, cannot be absorbed and serves as food for the microbial population in the gut. Too much lactose in the diet results in an overgrowth of fermenting bacteria and leads to stomach discomfort, gas, and diarrhea. Lactose products are milk, processed cheeses, commercial yogurts, and any other products that contain milk, nonfat dry milk, or whey (milk protein) as ingredients. However, it must be pointed out that some people are also sensitive or allergic to the whey protein structure of the milk and therefore lactose-free milk could still be a problem.

Natasha Campbell-McBride, MD, a neurologist and nutritionist in London, author of *Gut and Psychology Syndrome* (2004) and successor to Gottschall's work, does not allow any milk products in the first year of the diet because casein, the protein component of milk, in a compromised gut can lead to as many as thirty-three different neurological disorders. I think it okay to experiment with small amounts of rice milk or almond milk for a short time if a person is struggling to give up cow's milk.

Is the Diet Safe?

The diet has existed for more than sixty years with thousands of success stories associated with it. The SCD is far more nutritious than the standard American diet. The SCD is not an expensive drug. The largest costs are in time preparing foods, in cravings for favorite processed foods, and in expense of good-quality whole foods. Most people on the SCD find that better health is worth the effort. One could calculate *the money saved* from costly medical bills and productive hours lost to symptoms of the illness.

A popular complaint is "I could never live without [insert food here, such as pasta, corn, milk, bread, soda, etc]." However, the SCD offers a variety of substitutes that one will grow to love even more than one's current favorites. And some people will not live long or have quality of life unless they make the necessary dietary changes. "The Specific Carbohydrate Diet presented in this book is highly nutritious and well balanced. It is safe and very likely to be effective in overcoming many lingering and vexing intestinal and digestive problems" (Gottschall, 2007, p. 4). I have to agree!

I want to make clear that it is okay to use the gut medications that your doctors prescribe for the short term, but it's not recommended for the long term. From my own perspective, I used prescription medications for many years, got to a point of stability, and made changes in my diet, lifestyle, and attitude while reducing my dependency on the medications. Some seem to think it is "SCD or bust" in that prescription medication cannot be taken at all when doing the SCD. Gottschall wrote otherwise many times. Any weaning off of prescription medication must be done in conjunction with the physician who prescribed the drug. The SCD does not exclude medications or conventional treatments and does not carry dangerous side effects as some medications do.

As far as oral iron supplements, years of scientific research have shown these to aggravate bacterial infections. Anemia will be helped with ample servings of liver paté and animal products containing iron along with the vitamin supplements suggested in Gottscall's book. In fact, B_{12} shots are advisable with sufficient oral folic acid as these two supplements, especially, will help the anemia. Vitamin C will help iron absorption once the SCD heals the intestine.

What about Weight Gain?

For people who are underweight, as long as the gut symptoms are improving, weight gain will follow. After all, one could stuff 10,000 calories into a sick person without weight gain since absorption of calories and nutrients will not take place if the intestine is inflamed and subject to hypermotility because of a microbial infection. Once the intestine heals, digestion will proceed in a normal fashion and weight gain will likely follow if it is medically necessary.

Gottschall received many letters from people who had five feet or less of small intestine and barely any colon and then tried the SCD and recovered. The SCD does affect the absorption and transport across the gut mucosa. The diet repairs the microvilli that are involved with both. The SCD brings a highly acidic colon down to a normal pH balance.

Sweeteners and Fillers

Many ask why honey is permissible, but not other sugars like barley malt or molasses. Honey contains a single sugar and is assimilated directly into the bloodstream. Barley malt, molasses, and maple syrup are complex sugars and need to be broken down by enzymes or they will feed the pathogens.

From time to time people question whether various sweeteners and fillers are legal on the diet. In the following paragraphs are explanations of why they are not allowed. The Healing Crow website is my source for many of these.

Agave nectar is not made from the sap of the yucca or agave plant but from the starch of its giant pineapple-like root bulb. The principal constituent of the agave root is starch, similar to the starch in corn or rice, and a complex carbohydrate called inulin, which is made up of chains of fructose molecules. Technically a highly indigestible fiber, inulin, which does not taste sweet, comprises about half of the carbohydrate content of agave. Agave syrup is a manmade sweetener that has been through a complicated chemical refining process of enzymatic digestion that converts the starch and fiber into the unbound, manmade chemical fructose.

Maltodextrin is a breakdown product of the polysaccharide amylopectin and a waste product when glucose is made from corn. It requires an enzyme on the intestinal mucosa microvilli called isomaltase to break it down. Isomaltase is in short supply in healthy people. Maltodextrins overfeed bacteria in the lower small intestine and colon when isomaltase is insufficient. The patient may suffer a setback.

Whey protein is a waste product from cheese, an inferior protein because it contains so much of the complex carbohydrate lactose and one that is most likely to cause allergic reactions. The lactose causes bacteria to ferment it vigorously. It contains lactoalbumin, a highly antigenic protein, unlike casein, the protein in the curd part of milk.

Carrageenan, a seaweed derivative, is a gum that is used as a thickener or fat substitute. Evidence from animal models has demonstrated that degraded carrageenan causes ulcerations and malignancies in the gastrointestinal tract.

Carrageenan may be found in pudding, ice cream, yogurt, cottage cheese, processed meats, condensed milk, soy milk products, cosmetics, toothpaste, and room fresheners (Wolfson, 2008).

Many of the probiotic cultures we purchase contain fructooligosaccharides. Natasha Trenev in her book *Probiotics: Nature's Internal Healers* (1998) says:

> Fructooligosaccharides, known as FOS, are carbohydrates found naturally in certain plants, such as Jerusalem artichokes, onions, and bananas. However, a Japanese process turns white, bleached cane sugar, by the action of a fungal enzyme, into FOS—a sugar polymer that our bodies cannot digest.

It is digested in the colon by the bacteria and may, therefore, change the metabolic activity of the colon, resulting in abnormal functions. FOS stimulates the growth of *Klebsiella* and possibly other pathogenic organisms. In one study, *Klebsiella* has been associated with the autoimmune disease ankylosing spondylosis. Gottschall reported that on her visit to UK in 1997 to present her paper on celiac disease, a group of professors at one of the universities agreed with her that FOS also appeared to support *Clostridium dificile*. FOS is not allowed on the SCD.

Mannitol is a sugar alcohol; that is, it is derived from a sugar by reduction. Mannitol is commonly formed via the hydrogenation of fructose, which is formed from either starch or sugar. It causes diarrhea if used in the beginning of the diet and, later, if too much is used. It is SCD illegal.

The reason aspartame is SCD illegal is that it is normally packed with lactose. The lactose is not on the label of commercial aspartame products. Also, granulated aspartame is cut with *maltodextrin* to make it look and act more like sugar.

Stevia is not allowed, not because of its carbohydrate content, but because the glycosides in stevia mimic a hormone that may interfere with heart function. It has not been cleared because of safety concerns. Gottschall wrote to a listserv member: "Stevia has a molecular structure similar to a steroid and I prefer you not use it as it may have physiological effects that are unknown to you or to me."

Splenda can cause bowel problems. Splenda is a sucralose-based artificial sweetener derived from sugar. Splenda usually contains 95 percent dextrose and maltodextrin combined with a small amount of mostly indigestible sucralose.

Sucralose is a perverted form of sucrose exchanging some hydrogen with chlorine molecules so the body cannot utilize it as an energy source. However, even though the human body cannot break it down, bacteria can. Seth Barrows of the Healing Crow site did a literature review and found a few strains that have mutated to use sucralose as an energy source.

Saccharine can be found without lactose, maltodextrin, or other illegal fillers and it is not anything like a carbohydrate. It is SCD legal.

Vegetable glycerin is okay.

Final Thoughts on Sugar

Between 1970 and 2003, total per capita consumption of sugar and sweetener consumption rose by 19 percent in the United States, going from 119 pounds per capita in 1970 to 142 pounds per capita in 2003 (Farah and Buzby, 2005). Refined sugars are addicting. Gottschall wrote on the listserv: "If you want a slow death, consume most of your diet in refined sugar and flour. No way the caloric value can be transformed into cellular energy ATP—ADENOSINE TRIPHOSPHATE" (Gottschall, email, 8/31/01).

While Gottschall did her research on the effect of sugars on the gut wall, a group of other researchers were doing parallel research on sugar metabolism. Although Gottschall's original study was the effect of sugar on the gut wall especially as it caused IBD, IBS, and other autoimmune conditions, other authors have widened the net of what other conditions the complex sugars such as sucrose and high-fructose corn syrup (HFCS) can cause. John Yudkin, MD, PhD (1978) was one of the pioneer researchers examining the link between sugar and various degenerative illnesses. As far back as 1957 he showed that sugar consumption in England was more closely associated with coronary heart disease than the widely blamed saturated fats from animal foods.

The back cover of his book reads, "In this headline making book, Dr. John Yudkin, a renowned physician, biochemist, and researcher whose pioneering studies in sugar have been recognized throughout the world, offers never-before-published findings about sugar and explains, clearly and concisely, why ordinary table sugar is a critical health issues for all ages." Since 1957 he showed that the consumption of sugar and refined sweeteners is closely associated with coronary heart disease and type 2 diabetes. Studies he conducted on sugars and starches indicated that they raised blood triglycerides and insulin levels.

Robert H. Lustig, MD (2009) is a professor working in the University of California San Francisco (UCSF) Division of Endocrinology and Metabolism. As of July 23, 2011, more than a million and a half people have seen his educational and noncommercial YouTube video titled "Sugar: The Bitter Truth." Lustig describes himself as a "Yudkin acolyte" and says "every single thing this guy [Yudkin] has said has come to pass."

Lustig is also a Professor of Clinical Pediatrics at UCSF. He has authored more than eighty-five research articles and forty-five book chapters and is the former chairman of the Obesity Task Force of the Pediatric Endocrine Society, a member of the Obesity Task force of The Endocrine Society, and on the steering committee of the International Endocrine Alliance to Combat Obesity. He has become popular through his efforts to draw attention to the effects that the natural sugar fructose can have on human, especially children's, health if consumed in large amounts. In his YouTube lecture, Lustig notably calls fructose a "poison" and compares its metabolic effects with those of ethanol. He is particularly critical of the widespread use of high-fructose corn syrup in the United States.

With his special interest in childhood obesity, Lustig is concerned about the epidemic of obesity in six-month-old infants (Kim et al., 2006). He says that no child can choose to become obese, especially since its cause is from altered placental dynamics. He compared the contents of the infant formula Isomil by Similac to a Coca-Cola. The sugar contents are similar: 43.2 percent corn syrup solids and 10.3 percent sucrose. He says the earlier you introduce sugar to a person, in this case a baby, the greater will be the craving for it later. Isomil is like serving babies a big milkshake day after day, habituating them to sugar consumption.

Sugar in all its forms is a chronic toxin, not an acute toxin. As Lustig says, "it's not toxic after one meal but after 1,000 meals." What Lustig documents is that it's not the calories of sugar that are causing the big problem; it's how we metabolize sugar that is the culprit in so many chronic degenerative diseases. Fructose is metabolized by the liver, not by the whole body, as is sucrose. Hepatic fructose metabolism leads to all the manifestations of metabolic syndrome: hypertension, lipogenesis (fat formation), dyslipidemia (abnormal amounts of fats and/or cholesterol in the blood), NASH (nonalcoholic steatohepatitis), inflammation, hepatic insulin resistance, obesity, and central nervous system (CNS) leptin resistance promoting continuous consumption. Lustig calls fructose a chronic hepatotoxin, or "alcohol without the buzz."

Gary Taubes (2011) has spent the last decade doing journalistic research on diet and chronic disease. He concurs with Lustig that when the liver converts the fructose to fat it creates insulin resistance. The liver actually exports out free fatty acids that are taken into the cells and the fat in the cells prevents the acceptance of insulin. Even individual cells become obese. Insulin resistance is considered the fundamental problem in obesity and the underlying defect in heart disease and type 2 diabetes. He feels that it might also be the underlying defect in many human cancers.

In hepatic insulin resistance, the liver does not take up glucose or store it as glycogen in response to insulin. It leaks glucose into the blood stream in high amounts. This is attributed to fat being created and stored in the liver as a result of fructose metabolism. Both insulin and hepatic insulin resistance are caused by the same thing: too much fat being stored in the organ or cell driven by fructose metabolism, which leads to metabolic syndrome. According to Taubes, "physicians and medical authorities have come to accept the idea that a condition known as metabolic syndrome is a major, if not *the* major, risk factor for heart disease and diabetes." Include obesity in this group.

Melissa Diane Smith (2002, 2003) writes that a diet with refined carbohydrates is the biggest risk factor in diabetes. She attributes many conditions and complications to diabetes: polycystic ovary syndrome, amputations, blindness or retinopathy, complications in pregnancy, dental disease, heart disease and stroke, kidney damage or nephropathy, and nerve damage or neuropathy.

How does cancer fit into the sugar equation? Cancer is a disease that increases in incidence with obesity, diabetes, and metabolic syndrome according to the World Health Organization's International Agency for Research on Cancer in 2004. Taubes (2011) writes that cancer researchers report that insulin resistance leads the pancreas to secrete more insulin as well as a related hormone known as insulin-like growth factor that actually promotes tumor growth. The cells of many cancers eventually depend on insulin to provide the fuel, blood sugar, and materials they need to grow and multiply. Insulin and insulin-like growth factor and related growth factors also provide the signal for tumors to grow. Remember also the research that I cited in Chapter 2 regarding complex carbohydrates and cancer tumors.

Everyone in America is told by health care providers that the conditions associated with sugar consumption are preventable and controllable. However, part of the problem is the habituation or addiction individuals have to sugar. The challenge is to significantly fast oneself from the complex or highly refined carbohydrates and use instead the monosaccharides—the fruits, vegetables, honey, and homemade yogurt. Another part of the problem is that the government recommendations for daily sugar consumption are still too high according to a meta analysis of sugar research to be published in the fall of 2011.

> It is hoped that no one who recovers from his or her problem by following the SCD ever returns to a diet high in refined sugar and refined flours. These are lacking or low in nutrients, will not nourish the immune system adequately, and can make the individual more susceptible to intestinal infections.
>
> (Gottschall, 2007, p. 70)

Reprinted with permission from Sheila Shea. Quotes by Elaine Gottschall reprinted with permission.

CHAPTER 4

Comparison with Other
Diets and Conclusion

by Sheila Shea

I would like to compare a few other diets to the SCD. The most significant difference is that most other diets allow complex carbohydrates (grains).

Dr. Robert Atkins's *New Diet Revolution* (2002) has been on the bestseller list for many years. The Atkins diet initially dealt with weight loss and eventually encompassed heart disease and diabetes. He found that his patients all had a faulty carbohydrate metabolism. His prescribed diet drastically reduces the intake of any carbohydrate and focuses on proteins and fats. Atkins explained that the three monsters of cravings, fatigue, and hunger that accompany a high- or predominantly carbohydrate diet would disappear with extreme carbohydrate restriction. He mixed single and complex carbohydrates.

Eat Right for Your Type (D'Adamo, 1996) and *Live Right for Your Type* (D'Adamo and Whitney, 2000) point out some differences among blood types (O, A, B, AB) that dictate eating certain foods. Type O's diet appears to be that of the hunter-gatherers and Type O people do well with meat. Type As have a diet that is more like what we know as macrobiotics, with grain being the dietary base. I found some insight on the diet that guides me in making food choices and what I might avoid. It does include grain.

The Paleodiet described in Ray Audette's book *Neanderthin* (2000) focuses on a return to a diet followed long before concentrated agriculture of grains became predominant and people clustered in cities. The most nourishing diet is that of our hunter-gatherer ancestors—heavy on fruits and vegetables, supplemented by fish, lean meat, and nuts. "Cereal grains are what allowed us to leave the hunter-gatherer niche and form this vast cultural, technological society that we live in, yet there are many problems with cereal grains," said Dr. Loren Cordain, a professor at Colorado State University and a leading scholar of evo-

35

lutionary nutrition. For proponents of the Paleolithic diet, the chief pitfalls of the modern diet are its reliance on grains and some processed fats that are ill-suited to a genetic makeup little changed in thousands of years and the cause of modern illnesses. Beans and dairy are also not allowed. SCD allows some beans and dairy.

The Hellers published *The Carbohydrate Addict's Diet* (1993). Although I have not read the book, I do have a video of the show they did with Oprah and it is in the genre of low-carbohydrate diets. It does allow some grain. Gottschall commented on the theories of Allan and Lutz in their book *Life Without Bread* (2000) and the Hellers' suggested diet, along with many others. Gottschall disagreed with their insistence that all carbohydrate is digested into sugar, absorbed into the blood, and stimulates insulin production that they say is related to disease and obesity. Rather than the person ingesting all that starch and absorbing it into the bloodstream, Gottschall felt that the microbes are using it and the by-products of their metabolism create the problems.

The *Body Ecology Diet* by Donna Gates and Linda Schatz (2011) is designed with intestinal health in mind and contains wonderful information on liver support. However, the diet allows some grains. Dr. Crook's book *The Yeast Connection* (1986) is devoted strictly to candida. Dean Ornish's diet (1995) for heart disease is low-fat and high-carbohydrate.

In 1975, I was introduced to the raw vegan diet at Hippocrates Health Institute in Boston. Vegan means *no* animal products. Raw or living means *nothing* is cooked on this diet. It consists of fruits, vegetable, sprouts, nuts, seeds, wheat grass, and fermented foods. I recently heard a lecture by Paul Nison, author of *The Raw Life* (2000), on how he healed his ulcerative colitis using raw foods. Another branch of living foods includes eating raw animal products including organ meats and insects. These diets can be done with zero grains.

Vegetarian and nonraw vegan diets are popular. The vegetarian sometimes includes dairy products. Very often, these two diets include a predominance of grain, soy, and starchy roots. I have been reading two other books with information on gut health. One is by Scala, *The New Eating Right For a Bad Gut* (2000), and the other by Patel-Thompson, *Listen to Your Gut* (2006). Both allow grains.

It's possible to learn something from each book that would provide an intestinal health insight. However, the point of reviewing the various diets is to show the treatment of grains and complex sugars by each system.

When Do I Begin?

Many timing issues come up when we undertake a new diet or practice. When do I begin? When do I introduce certain foods? The gut wall has to heal to a certain degree to allow some of the more complex foods such as the beans or cheeses. A person who has diabetes or candida might have to temper the single sugars initially until the intestines or pancreas are more stable or balanced and the positive bacteria more in charge. When a flareup happens, what is the best course of action? The road to health is not a straight line from A to Z. It has zigs and zags along the way. Sometimes one has to retreat to the beginning levels of the diet, or leave out some offending food for the time being, or test for food sensitivity. So much of the timing has to do with the level of the healing of the gut wall.

The *basic idea* is to end the bacterial and fungal destruction of the intestinal wall by depriving bacteria and fungus of the foods that give them energy. It takes time for the microvilli of the small intestine to repair themselves. Gottschall said that after one heals the small or large intestinal track and has *no symptoms for one year*, one can slowly introduce grains, potatoes, yams, pasta, and soy products. At that point, I would recommend getting tested for food sensitivities and allergies regarding gluten, dairy, and soy. Some people find they can never return to complex carbohydrates.

Strict adherence is necessary to obtain relief from symptoms. Thirty days is the initial time suggested to test the diet. People with IBD often note significant improvement in their symptoms within three weeks of starting the Gottschall diet. By twelve weeks, the majority are recovering definitively. One twenty-year-old patient of Dr. Hoffman with ulcerative colitis took a full year to become symptom-free. Another patient of his with ulcerative proctitis affecting the rectum had daily bloody diarrhea despite medications for years until initiating the SCD. After eighteen months, he became completely symptom-free without the aid of medications. Dr. Haas has a chart in his book (Haas and Haas, 1951, p. 145) showing that eighteen to twenty-four months is the time when most people experience recovery. A few individuals take up to four years.

One person revealed that she had a very weak digestion and originally did better with pure protein, fat, or fat with protein. After almost a year and a half on the diet, she can eat some beans such as lentils and it feels very nourishing. Gottschall said on the listserv: "It depends on where you are at with your condition. Four days is just not time enough to expect the diet to kick in although it has happened in neurological problems like seizures in children. It will take longer, perhaps three weeks, before I would expect a change in the diarrhea."

People ask why the diet is not working for them when it is working for many others. Gottschall admitted she did not know the answer and suggested getting a test for *Clostridium dificile. C. dificile,* an antibiotic-caused bacterium, has been found in and infected almost all cases of a relapse in ulcerative colitis (UC) after a long period of improvement on the SCD. When testing positive, their doctor puts them on a regimen usually prescriptive. After taking the regimen of the doctor, they continue to follow the diet and most continue to improve. Gottschall counseled that 25 percent of UC patients are not helped by the diet.

Generally, a resection of the stomach is required when people go on the SCD and are still prone to blockages such as the narrowing of the intestines that cannot be reversed by diet alone. However, the blockages can be prevented from occurring again using the diet. Peristalsis, or the contractions and relaxations that are a normal part of intestinal movement, cannot occur when inflammation at the ileum or another part of the small intestine destroys the elastic fibers of the muscle wall of the small intestine. In this case, the intestine narrows and it has no elasticity to expand itself. We call this loss of elasticity and the narrowing of the lumen by the thickening of the walls fibrosis. As a result, certain foods like raw fruits and vegetables such as grated cabbage and carrots, even raw pears and apples, may plug the gut. The SCD does not reverse the fibrosis. Some who have come to the diet have had a resection. Others have existing fibrosed walls that might require a resection. However, future blockages can be prevented from occurring again using the diet. The SCD prevents the gut wall from further inflammation and fibrosis.

Gottschall believed that the number of causative microorganisms such as mutated bacteria and various pathological yeasts decrease in number after a person is on the SCD for a period of time and recovering because of avoiding complex sugars. Very often a flu virus, respiratory infection, or the emergence from a *hibernated* state brings about a flare. The person goes to the doctor, who treats them with a combination of antibiotics and prescription Flagyl, and the few remaining pathogens are wiped out. Gottschall felt that sometimes time and patience might have the same result, although it takes longer and is more stressful.

What Else Is There to Eat?

I get this question from some people after I tell them about the SCD. I know right away what their diet is! Clearly for them no foods exist other than complex carbohydrates. Politically, it could be called an "isolationist" diet: It's just me and my carbs and no other food group exists unless it enhances my first love, carbohydrate. Pizza, bread, and ice cream are the big examples here.

For some, eliminating or restricting the complex carbohydrates in their diet is just too overwhelming. Our culture fosters the overindulgence or overeating of carbohydrates more than any other food category, even protein. One of my clients made an affirmative statement about the SCD after following it faithfully for a few months. She noted that she no longer feels the food cravings and unexplained hunger that she used to have. Now that's an incentive. Other factors influence our ability to find intestinal health through diet. One is our biochemical individuality, our enterotype as noted in an earlier chapter, and, finally, our ability to accept responsibility for our health.

Each of us is unique in our chemical composition and it's important to stay in touch with our instinct and intuition as we proceed. This requires more body awareness to sensations in the gut especially. For example, many people tend to ignore signals for the need to evacuate the bowel. It also means to slow down and eat mindfully. Making dietary shifts for any reason seems to be very difficult for some people. Many people are compensating for other problems in their life with a bad or simply a convenient diet of mainly fast food. Some claim to not have the time to make better choices.

So, the buck stops with you and me. I have to be willing to take responsibility for my choices, my behavior changes, and being in the driver's seat on the journey to gut health. This involves a commitment to take care of myself and forgive myself for relapses or past mistakes. As I said at the very beginning, self-regulation is critical for survival and freedom. And self-regulation takes time and getting help from other people as necessary.

A Few Final Thoughts

Gottschall commented on two types of individuals that have adopted the diet. Some stay on the diet, following it about 85 percent of the time, and remain well. Others go off the deep end and return to a junk food diet and get sick again. She said that people will stay healthy and well as long as they use intelligence in making their dietary choices. Intelligence is clearly on the 85-percent side. The diet gives people remission of their symptoms as well as a guide to eating, which when remission is achieved, prevents further occurrence of the disease. Gottschall felt that when people are educated to know what foods are compatible with their biological makeup they can be free of digestive problems that she believed are caused by economic and political agendas.

I have taken the reader through a long exploration of conditions, causes, and dietary specifics. I am sure many questions remain: How do I do it? How can I give up all the goodies? How can I make something? I don't have time—will I ever succeed? How will I do it at work? What do I eat for breakfast? How long do I stay on the introductory diet? When do I go back to it? What do I need to do if I continue to lose weight? Will the diet help me lose weight? What happens when I get a flareup? Find help in your community and read the books cited and look at the resources I have provided below. Educating one's self is the first priority. Start slowly with one or two food items rather than an immediate complete overhaul. Be kind to yourself and your body. This is a diet of kindness. I support each person to do your best to make the necessary dietary changes that build intestinal health.

Some Definitions

Adenosine-5'-triphosphate (ATP) is a multifunctional nucleotide used in cells as a coenzyme. It is often called the molecular unit of currency of intracellular energy transfer. ATP transports chemical energy within cells for metabolism.

Arthralgia is severe pain in a joint.

A biofilm forms when bacteria adhere to a wet surface such as the gastrointestinal tract, and underlies many chronic diseases and infections. When a cell attaches to a surface, it expresses a different set of genes than it did originally and becomes, effectively, a significantly different organism. As such, bacteria can be almost impossible to eradicate with conventional antibiotics.

Candida is a naturally occurring fungus in the intestines that may grow out of control due to antibiotics, steroids, birth control pills, and/or the inability to metabolize complex sugars. Gottschall said that if one has a fungus overgrowth one has a bacterial overgrowth as they piggy-back on each other. Both the pathogenic bacteria and fungi give off toxic metabolites that affect the integrity of the gut wall. In this way, IBD and candida are related.

Celiac disease is an inflammatory bowel disease, an autoimmune disorder of the small intestine that occurs in genetically predisposed people of all ages from middle infancy onward. Symptoms include chronic diarrhea, failure to thrive in children, migraine, dermatitis herpetiformis, and fatigue. Symptoms may be absent or may occur in other organ systems. Gottschall theorized that the cause lies in complex sugars, and I agree. Others theorize that the prolamins, plant storage proteins such as gluten, found in some grains—wheat, rye, barley, corn, and oats—are the cause. Research is being done now to distinguish between gluten sensitivity and celiac. Regardless, the inflammatory reaction can ultimately lead to villous atrophy, a truncating of the villi that line the small intestines. The blunting, truncating, or damaging of the villi interferes with the absorption of nutrients because the intestinal villi are responsible for absorption.

Chronic diarrhea is the passage of fluid or unformed stool that lasts at least four weeks. In *Breaking the Vicious Cycle* (2007), Gottschall listed chronic diarrhea as an inflammatory bowel disease in and of itself. Chronic diarrhea may also be a symptom of other chronic diseases of the intestines such as irritable bowel syndrome, celiac disease, or Crohn's. Causes are bacterial, viral, or parasitic. Chronic diarrhea symptoms may be continual or they may come and go.

Crohn's disease is an inflammatory bowel disease marked by patchy areas of full-thickness inflammation anywhere in the gastrointestinal tract, from mouth to anus. It frequently involves the terminal ileum of the small intestine or the proximal large intestine and may be responsible for abdominal pain, diarrhea, malabsorption, fistula formation between the intestines and other organs, and bloody stools. It also is called granulomatous enteritis or colitis, regional enteritis, ileitis, or terminal ileitis. Crohn's disease may cause complications outside the gastrointestinal tract such as skin rashes, arthritis, inflammation of the eye, fatigue, and lack of concentration.

Constipation is a decrease in the frequency of passage of formed stools and is characterized by stools that are hard and difficult to pass. This definition suggests four characteristics that may be presented in the acronym DISH: difficult to pass, infrequent compared to normal, smaller than normal, and hard (McMillan, 2004).

Cystic fibrosis (CF) is an inherited disease of the secretory glands such as the glands that make mucus and sweat. The name *cystic fibrosis* refers to the characteristic scarring (fibrosis) and cyst formation within the pancreas. Cystic fibrosis mainly affects the lungs, pancreas, liver, intestines, sinuses, and sex organs. Our focus here is the intestines, liver, and pancreas. With CF, mucus becomes thick and sticky and may block the biliary ducts of the liver and the pancreatic ducts of the pancreas, hence preventing digestive enzymes of these organs from reaching the small intestines. Malnutrition and vitamin deficiency may result. Other symptoms may be bulky stools, intestinal gas, a swollen belly from severe constipation, pain or discomfort, and an abnormally high electrolyte concentration in the sweat. Complications resulting from CF might be pancreatitis, rectal prolapse, liver disease due to inflamed or blocked bile ducts, diabetes, or gallstones, according to the National Institutes of Health website.

Dermatitis herpetiformis (DH) or Duhring's disease is a chronic blistering skin condition characterized by blisters filled with a watery fluid. Despite its name, DH is not related to or caused by the herpes virus; the name means that it is a skin inflammation having an appearance similar to herpes. Dermatitis herpetiformis is characterized by intensely itchy, chronic, pimple-like blister eruptions usually distributed symmetrically on extensor surfaces (buttocks, back of neck, scalp, elbows, knees, back). The blisters vary in diameter up to 1 cm across.

Diverticulitis is the condition of the diverticula, small pockets or pouches that branch off from the gut wall, becoming infected and developing abscesses or even perforating. Pain is a major symptom.

Diverticulosis is the condition of having diverticula in the colon that are out-pocketings of the colonic mucosa and submucosa through weaknesses of muscle layers in the colon wall. The diverticula are like aneurysms of the gut wall. They are more common in the sigmoid colon, a common place for increased pressure. The diverticula may bleed, rapidly causing bleeding through the rectum or slowly causing anemia. Other symptoms of diverticulosis are cramps and tenderness in the affected areas, bloating, alternating diarrhea or constipation, nonspecific chronic discomfort in the lower left abdomen with occasional acute episodes of sharper pain, and abdominal pain in the left lower abdomen often after meals.

Erythema is a reddening of the outer skin of the body or the inner skin that we call the gut wall, usually found in patches. Dilation of the superficial blood vessels in the gut wall causes erythema.I consider it to be a precursor of inflammation of the bowel walls. Erythema is seen in numerous endoscopies and colonoscopies.

Fibrin is a white filamentous protein involved in the final stage of blood clotting.

A ganglion is a mass of nerve cell bodies. Cells found in a ganglion are called ganglion cells.

Gluten is a protein present in practically all grains in one form or another. In wheat it encases the starch granule. In manufacturing cornstarch, gluten removal from the starch is an expensive process because the gluten is really stuck onto the starch.

Hirshsprung's disease is a blockage of the large intestine due to improper muscle movement in the bowel. It is a congenital condition, which means it is present from birth. Muscle contractions in the gut help digested materials move through the intestine. This is called peristalsis. Nerves between the muscle layers trigger the contractions. In Hirschsprung's disease, the nerves are missing from a part of the bowel. Areas without such nerves cannot push material through. This causes a blockage. Intestinal contents build up behind the blockage, causing the bowel and abdomen to become swollen.

Inflammatory bowel disease (IBD) is a set of inflammatory diseases of the intestines including Crohn's disease, ulcerative and mucus colitis, chronic diarrhea, diverticulosis and diverticulitis, celiac disease, and cystic fibrosis.

Irritable bowel syndrome (IBS) is a syndrome characterized by abdominal pain often relieved by the passage of stool or gas. IBS is characterized by disturbances of evacuation such as constipation, diarrhea, or alternating constipation and diarrhea, as well as bloating and abdominal distention, and the passage of mucus in the stool. These symptoms must be present despite the absence of anatomical, biochemical, or clinical evidence of other active intestinal diseases. In some individuals, IBS may have an acute onset and develop after an infectious illness characterized by two or more of the following: fever, vomiting, diarrhea, or positive stool culture. This postinfective syndrome has consequently been termed "postinfectious IBS." The symptoms of IBS occur more often in patients who have a history of physical or sexual abuse in childhood than in patients without such a history.

Leptin is a protein hormone manufactured primarily in the adipocytes of white adipose tissue that plays a key role in regulating energy intake and energy expenditure, including appetite and metabolism. Leptin acts on receptors in the hypothalamus of the brain where it inhibits appetite. Fructose metabolism bypasses the brain.

Meconium is the earliest stools of an infant. Unlike later feces, meconium is composed of materials ingested during the time the infant spends in the uterus: intestinal epithelial cells, lanugo, mucus, amniotic fluid, bile, and water. Meconium is almost sterile, unlike later feces; it is viscous and sticky like tar, and has no odor. It should be completely passed by the end of the first few days of life, with the stools progressing toward yellow (digested milk).

Mucus colitis is an inflammatory bowel disease of the mucous membrane of the colon characterized by colicky pain, intestinal spasms, constipation or diarrhea, and the passage of mucous or slimy pseudomembranous shreds and patches. It is also called myxomembranous colitis and is characterized by the passage of unusually large amounts of mucus.

Nucleotides are molecules that, when joined together, make up the structural units of RNA and DNA. In addition, nucleotides play central roles in metabolism.

Planktonic cell are individual cells in a laboratory setting rather than cells that can intermingle with a medium such as the gut, prosthetic devices, and teeth to which they can adhere to form a biofilm.

A pseudomembrane is a leaf- or shelf-like exudate made of inflammatory debris and fibrin that may form on the epithelial or cell wall surfaces of the intestines.

Short stature in celiac. Children with celiac often do not grow according to their age and remain shorter and smaller than other children their age.

Steatohepatitis is a type of liver disease characterized by inflammation of the liver with concurrent fat accumulation in liver ("steato," meaning fat; "hepatitis," meaning inflammation of the liver). Classically seen in alcoholics as part of alcoholic liver disease, steatohepatitis also is frequently found in people with diabetes and obesity. When not associated with excessive alcohol intake, it is referred to as nonalcoholic steatohepatitis, or NASH, and is the progressive form of the relatively benign nonalcoholic fatty liver disease. Steatohepatitis of either etiology may progress to cirrhosis, and NASH is now believed to be a frequent cause of unexplained cirrhosis (at least in Western societies).

Stomatitis is inflammation of the mucous membrane of the mouth.

Ulcerative colitis (UC) is an inflammatory bowel disease marked pathologically by continuous inflammation of the intestinal mucosa that typically involves the anus, rectum, and distal colon and sometimes affects the entire large intestine. Inflammation and ulcers typically affect only the innermost lining in these areas compared with the deeper lesions seen in Crohn's disease. According to Tabor's Cyclopedic Medical Dictionary (Venes, 2009), ulcerative colitis is associated with an increased incidence of cancer of the colon.

Urticaria is another name for hives that are raised, often itchy, red welts on the surface of the skin.

SCD Resources

www.breakingtheviciouscycle.info Official site for the SCD. You can do an Amazon search to read the many testimonials from readers of the book.

www.scdrecipe.com A good site with recipes.

www.scdiet.org/3testimonials/perspective.htm One person's exciting story and good links on the SCD.

www.scdiet.net/healingcrow/HealingCrow/www.healingcrow.com/index.html The Healing Crow site was taken down, but John Chalmers from SCdiet.net archived the information before the site went under. One of the top resource sites for SCD and IBD help.

www.drhoffman.com/page.cfm/787 Book of recipes for SCD by Sandra Ramacher, Foreword by Ronald Hoffman, MD.

www.drhoffman.com/page.cfm/170 Here you can read Dr. Hoffman's update on inflammatory bowel disease.

www.ibduk.com IBD and Crohn's disease information site in the UK.

pecanbread.com Kids and SCD (listserv available).

www.scdiet.org/7archives/crohnsref.html Source of scientific research on scdiet.org site.

www.scdiet.org SCD web library. Excellent research articles.

Reprinted with permission from Sheila Shea. Quotes by Elaine Gottschall reprinted with permission.

SECTION II

. . .

Biodynamic Practice

CHAPTER 5

The Zones of Perception

These zones are convenient metaphors for describing how a practitioner moves her perception during a session. Zones are boundaries of awareness that gradually disappear during a session, leaving a single continuum of perception. The practitioner moves her attention between the zones, sensing the rhythmic balanced interchange of Primary Respiration and stillness. The *heart-midline* as used here represents the focal point of this interchange. The zones should be thought of as a container. It is the responsibility of the practitioner to build a safe container in order for Primary Respiration to manifest its healing potencies.

The basic unit of perceptual work in a biodynamic session is called a *cycle of attunement.* This is how the practitioner builds the container for transformation. The process of a cycle of attunement requires the practitioner to move her attention from zone A to zone D and back to A deliberately in the tempo of Primary Respiration. Gradually, this deliberate movement of attention becomes spontaneous. Further, the use of embryonic and fetal metaphors to define the various spaces of the zones as a biological reality is quite handy in a clinical context. Since the therapeutic relationship is a two-person biology, these developmental metaphors become a living reality containing therapeutic significance for optimal outcomes in the treatment.

I like to use these metaphors as teaching protocols in my classes. I ask the students to form groups of three and four and to assume the various embryonic and fetal spaces as shown in this chapter. For example, the client on the table becomes the embryo, the practitioner becomes the chorion with the hands and arms being a connecting stalk, the third person becomes the uterus, and so forth. These exercises are all done within the perception of the balanced, rhythmic interchange of Primary Respiration and stillness. Once the practitioner is alone with the client in clinical practice, it is not unusual at all to experience this type of morphology in the practitioner's body, the client's body, and the space of the office and natural world. As a note of caution, one should not overuse these metaphors in clinical practice, but rather allow them to spontaneously emerge or use them briefly to evaluate the availability of an ignition for healing.

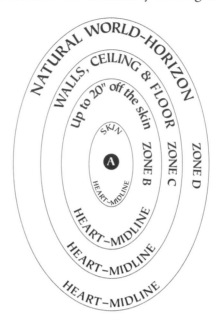

Figure 5.1. Zones of perception

The zones are one integrated continuum or container. Dashed lines in Figure 5.2 indicate permeable boundaries between the zones. One could add a fourth fulcrum based on embryology to zone A. That fourth fulcrum would be the bladder or, as it is called in embryology, the allantois. Of particular clinical interest is the way in which zones A and B form an integrated whole or container for several aspects of the Mid Tide or the potency of Primary Respiration. For example, the longitudinal fluctuation ascends from the coccyx up to the third ventricle and cascades out into zone B to recoalesce at the coccyx at the end of one cycle. Likewise, the reciprocal tension potency is a three-dimensional pulse emanating from the embryonic midline of the body as it extends out into zone B. The clinical relevance of this cannot be underestimated. The practitioner must maintain awareness of his or her own integrated space of zones A and B and that of the client when working biodynamically. Of course, such awareness is not an object of focus for the entire session, but rather an awareness that is periodically revisited in the cycle of attunement. The awareness of zones A and B begins with sensing the stillness in both while maintaining attention on the surface of the skin or zone A of the practitioner. From this perspective the practitioner can observe how his or her zones A and B fill up with the potencies of Primary Respiration.

In addition, measurements of the electromagnetic field coming from the human heart made by the Institute of HeartMath have indicated that the human heart can have an effect out to zones C and D. Thus it could be inferred that all of the zones are an effect of the human heart. Once again, the zones provide a convenient metaphor for exploring the container of the therapeutic process.

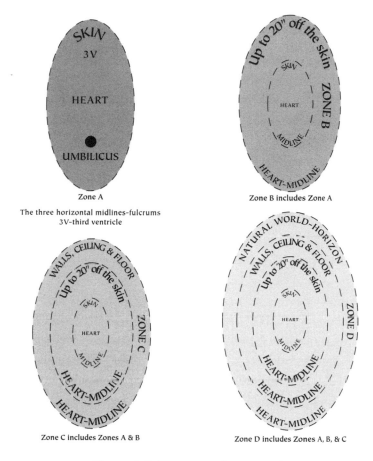

Figure 5.2. The zones integrated

Figure 5.3 on epigenesis begins exploring another metaphor for the zones. It is an embryonic metaphor related to the metabolic fields of the embryo. Research indicates that genetic imprinting on the ovum starts in our great grandparents when they were adolescents and reflects traumatic stress. Furthermore, during prenatal development, the fetus has distinct genes that need to be activated. Some of these genes in the embryo and fetus are from the mother. Likewise, there are important genes in the placenta from the father. Maternal stress interferes with the proper genetic expression of both the mother's genes in the embryo and fetus and the father's genes in the placenta.

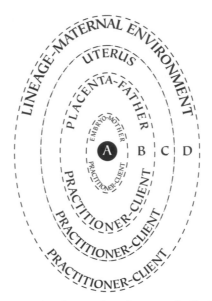

Figure 5.3. The zones and epigenesis—the metabolic fields of the embryo

The next figure on epigenesis, Figure 5.4, shows the application of the zones of perception in biodynamic practice. It depicts pre-conception work, which is sensing ovum to ovum as an active visualization and a sensory reality by the practitioner. Neurological research indicates that a part of the human brain is monitoring this space. The practitioner periodically attempts to perceive zone B to zone B. Hands may make contact with the client zone A to zone A and thus go through zone B. This practice is especially valuable for clients with hypersensitive autonomic nervous systems. Zone C must be still. The practitioner focuses on the stillness in zone B as the starting point.

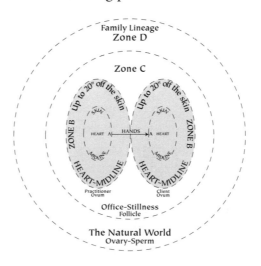

Figure 5.4. Working zone B to zone B

The zones represent another important biodynamic principle: the therapeutic relationship is a two-person biology based on pre- and perinatal metabolism. It is called the Law of Exchange. *Metabolism* as used here means the physical or biokinetic metabolic movements of the whole rather than the chemistry of the fluids. The practitioner–client relationship is like a circulatory system in which the practitioner and client exchange roles via the cardiovascular system during a session. In other words, the practitioner and client periodically trade places among the zones as if mirroring embryonic development. This perceptual experience is managed by the practitioner's somatic awareness. Figure 5.5 depicts the early conceptus after fertilization in which the different functional components of the conceptus are indicated. These metaphors for the therapeutic relationship become alive when the practitioner perceives Primary Respiration.

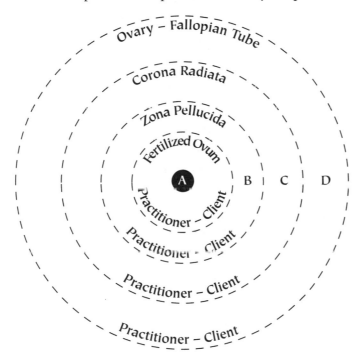

Figure 5.5. The zones as the conceptus

Figure 5.6 depicts another prenatal metaphor regarding the practitioner–client exchange. This is the embryonic time in general. Any metabolism in one zone can automatically exchange function with another zone between the practitioner and client. The therapeutic relationship is in constant flux. Through the use of creative visualization and sensing Primary Respiration, the practitioner and client can experience any of the fluid cavity dynamics while the practitioner's arms and hands act like a connecting stalk.

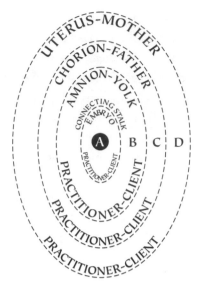

Figure 5.6. The zones as the embryo

Figure 5.7 is more directly related to fetal development and thus the exchange between the fetus and mother (client-practitioner or vice versa). Here the focus is on the movement of the heart in the practitioner, because the therapeutic relationship is an interpersonal cardiovascular system. The therapeutic relationship depends on the practitioner's perception and attention, which often fluctuates within the fluid body of both the practitioner and client and out to nature and back in the tempo of Primary Respiration. The container must be flexible and capable of expanding to include the whole pregnancy.

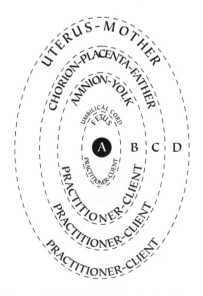

Figure 5.7. The zones as the fetus

With an understanding of the zones as presented, now the practitioner can practice as depicted in Figure 5.8, in a cycle of attunement in which the practitioner moves her attention between zone A and D and back. As depicted here, the first four steps only involve the practitioner. Steps 5 through 7 involve the practitioner's perception of self and client. Zone B to zone B requires repeated attempts and multiple sessions to establish prenatal and pre-conception resonance. This is a nonlinear sequence in which the practitioner waits for a stillness to permeate the office space and then focuses on her zone B, followed by that of the client. It is basically two eggs meeting at their borders while the practitioner senses Primary Respiration breathing both eggs or one or the other, all the while being held by the stillness of zone C.

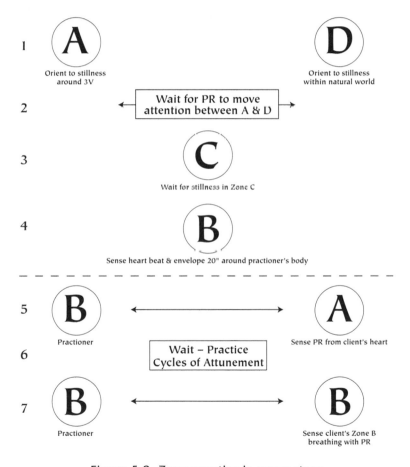

Figure 5.8. Zone practice in seven steps

CHAPTER 6

Definition of Attunement by Leading Researchers and Clinicians

The intention of this series of passages from four books, and related research on attention and nature, is to support full understanding of *attunement* as it relates to biodynamic practice. In the literature used as the basis for this chapter, attunement is also referred to as *affect attunement.* I have divided this chapter into four sections, starting with infant-mother attunement, followed by adult-adult attunement, then research on attention to nature, and closing with attention to zone B around the body.

Affect attunement at a biodynamic level of understanding means to be not only able to attune to one's self and the client but also to the space immediately around the practitioner's and client's bodies, to the office space, and to nature and then back cyclically. It involves the spontaneous and deliberate movement of attention between these boundaries of awareness very slowly and the simultaneous capacity to be still or rest one's attention on one's heart and breathing. Affect attunement practiced in this way builds resonance, empathy, and compassion. Consequently, the principle therapeutic affect that a biodynamic practitioner seeks to attune with is love. This is done by starting with an orientation to stillness in self and other and the subsequent perception of the interchange between stillness and Primary Respiration.

All quoted material is reprinted with permission.

Research on Infant Attunement

Daniel Stern's book *The Present Moment in Psychotherapy and Everyday Life* (Stern, 2004) is the source for the extracted quotations in this section on infant-mother attunement. The references cited are Stern's, and they are included in the bibliography of this book.

From Stern's definition of attunement in his glossary:

Affect attunement (also attunement) is a special form of behavior in response to the communicative affective behavior of another. Just as imitation is a faithful rendering of the other's overt actions, affect attunement is a faithful rendering of what the other must have felt like when he or she expressed him- or herself with those actions. This requires that the attunement imitates only the temporal dynamics of the intensity, form, or rhythm of the other's behavior but in a different modality or at a different scale. In this way, the actual actions of the other do not become the referent of the attunement (as they would for imitation); rather, the feeling behind the actions becomes the referent. It is a way of imitating, from the inside, what an experience feels like, not how it was expressed in action.

(p. 241)

From Stern's text:

My colleagues and I have taken a third route (Stern, 1977, 1985, 2000; Stern et al., 1984). I have been more interested in how the dyad lets each other know about their inner feeling states. For instance, if an infant emitted an affective behavior after an event, how could the mother let the infant know that she grasped not simply what the infant did but also the feeling the infant experienced that lay behind what he did? The emphasis has shifted from the overt behavior to the subjective experience underlying it. I proposed *affect attunement,* a form of selective and cross-modal imitation, as the path to sharing inner feeling states, in contrast to faithful imitation as the path to sharing overt behavior....

The issue of coordinated timing is obviously central for synchronicity and the access to another's experience. Watson (1994) and Gergely and Watson (1999) have found a fascinating way that the infant becomes sensitive to the behavior and timing of others. They propose that we, and infants, have "innate contingency detection analyzers." Such modules measure the extent to which someone's behavior is exactly synchronous or responsive with your own. They find that before 3 months, infants are most interested in events that are perfectly contingent with their behavior. This would make babies most sensitive to themselves. Between 4 and 6 months there is a shift. Infants become most interested in events that are highly but imperfectly contingent with their own behavior. That is exactly what an interacting other person does. They now become most interested in the behavioral timing of others, using themselves as the standard.

The work of many others also bears significantly on these issues (e.g.:

Emde and Sorce, 1983; Klinnert et al., 1983; Sander, 1975, 1977, 1995; Stern, 1971; Stern and Gibbon, 1978; Tronick, 1989; Tronick, Als, and Adamson, 1979; Tronick, Als, and Brazelton, 1977). Most significant, all of these authors agreed that infants are born with minds that are especially attuned to other minds as manifested through their behavior. This is based in large part on the detection of correspondences in timing, intensity, and form that are intermodally transposable. The result is that from birth on, one can speak of a psychology of mutually sensitive minds.

(pp. 84–85)

Beatrice Beebe (with coauthors Stephen Knoblauch, Judith Rustin, and Dorienne Sorter), in *Intersubjectivity in Infant Research and Adult Treatment* (Beebe et al., 2005), couched their perspective on infant-mother attunement as intersubjectivity.

Stern, similar to Trevarthen, uses timing, form, and intensity to define the dimensions of correspondences. Stern is interested in the *how* of behavior, the dynamic, shifting patterns of rhythms, shapes, and activation. "Dynamic micro-momentary shifts in intensity over time that are perceived as patterned changes within ourselves and others" allow us, rather automatically and without awareness, to "change with" the other, to "feel-what-has-been-perceived-in-the-other" (Stern et al., 1985, p. 263)....

Stern defines three forms of intersubjectivity: joint attention, joint intention, and joint affect ("interaffectivity"). In describing joint *attention,* Stern notes that the infant's capacity to point and to follow the other's line of regard has been suggested by Brunner (1977) to constitute a critical means by which the infant can transcend egocentrism. In Emde's social referencing experiments, the infant is enticed by interesting toys to cross a glass table that is made to look like a "visual cliff." Infants hesitate, look back to mother, and cross only if mother's face indicates that it is safe. Stern suggests that this experiment portrays the infant's deliberate attempt to make sure that the focus of attention is being shared.

In describing joint *intention,* Stern is influenced by the work of Bates (1979, p. 36), who defined intentional communication as "signaling behavior in which the sender is aware, a priori, of the effect that the signal will have on his listener, and he persists in that behavior until the effect is obtained or failure is clearly indicated" (quoted by Stern, 1985, p. 130)....

Of the three forms of intersubjectivity, joint affect, or "affect attunement," is the first and most important mode of sharing subjective experiences. Throughout the first year, affects are both the "primary medium and the primary subject of communication" (Stern, 1985, p. 133)....

What is Stern's evidence for affect attunement? Nine- to twelve-month infants were videotaped in the lab during a free-play session with their mothers. Coders first noted moments whenever the infant made some affect expression—facial, vocal, gestural, or postural. Coders then evaluated the mother's observable response, for verbal comments, imitations (defined as matching within the same modality), and attunements (defined as matching across modalities). Attunements were coded along the dimensions of matching: intensity, timing, and shape of the infant's behavior. Note that these dimensions are identical to those of interest to Trevarthen. Intensity was subdivided into absolute intensity and intensity contour (acceleration/deceleration). Timing was subdivided into beat (a regular pulsation is matched), rhythm (a pattern of pulsations of unequal stress is matched), and duration. Shape was illustrated by the infant's up-down movement of the arm matched by the mother's up-down movements of the head.

The first finding was that, of all mother's responses, 33 percent were verbal comments, 19 percent were exact imitations of the infant's behavior, and 48 percent were considered attunements (occurring on average approximately once per minute). [This is Primary Respiration!] Second, in most attunements, more than one dimension of behavior was matched. Third, the dimension of intensity contour (profile of change in intensity over time) was the most frequent dimension of matching, occurring in 97 percent of attunements, and the dimension of timing the next most frequent, occurring in 76 percent....

These data together with his earlier work on younger infants (Stern, 1971; Stern, 1977), consolidated one of Stern's most central contributions, that is, his emphasis on the micromomentary dynamic shifts in each person's behavior that allow the partner to *change with* the other. Affect attunement is thus defined as the crossmodal matching of intensity, timing, and "shape" (contour) of behavior, based on dynamic micromomentary shifts over time, perceived as patterns of change that are similar in self and other. The infant perceives a mental state in the other, based on the intensity, timing, and shape of the partner's behavior. Stern argued that the infant's capacity to recognize crossmodal correspondences is the perceptual underpinning of affect attunement, enabling the infant to capture the quality of another's inner feeling state, and to discriminate whether it is shared.

Stern's description of affect attunements as "automatic," with relative lack of awareness, places them clearly within implicit, procedural processing. [In biodynamic practice, we are seeking to have attunement become conscious, which adds empathy, and thus, biodynamic practice becomes a protocol for compassion.]...

In discussing the possible functions of attunements, Stern differentiates between communication and communion. Examples of the functions of communication include: to imitate, to tune the baby up or down, to restructure the interaction, to reinforce, or to teach. Communing is something very different, to participate, to *share without altering,* to maintain the thread of feeling-connectedness. Affect attunement is a form of communing....

Stern described the two styles as attuning to enthusiasm vs. "exthusiasm." Each style, when exaggerated, can introduce a selective bias, placing the opposite pole outside the "shareable universe."

It is important to note that Stern does not consider affect attunement equivalent to empathy, although both concepts share the phenomenon of emotional resonance. Whereas attunement occurs largely automatically and out of awareness, empathy requires the mediation of cognitive processes (see Basch, 1977). "Attunement is a distinct form of affective transaction in its own right" (Stern, 1985, p. 145) and need not proceed toward empathic knowledge.

Unlike imitation, attunement shifts the focus to the quality of feeling that is "behind" the behavior. It treats the feeling quality as the referent, and the overt behavior as one of several possible expressions of the referent. "Attunement takes the experience of emotional resonance and recasts that experience into another form of expression," by way of nonverbal metaphor and analogy (Stern, 1985, p. 161). For example, the same level of exuberance might be expressed as a facial expression, a vocalization, or a gesture. All three overt behaviors would refer to the same inner state.

(pp. 44–48)

Continuing in Beebe et al.:

... the origin of mind begins at birth with the perception, "you are like me." The key mechanism is the perception and production of similarity. The sense of self derives from one's own movements as seen in the actions of the other, and actions of the other experienced proprioceptively as similar to one's own movements....

Stern emphasizes that the infant has a theory of *separate* minds. Two separate minds align to a third thing, an inner feeling state. The key mechanism of this alignment is a process of matching in which each partner is "changing with" the other. The crossmodal matching of form, timing, and intensity allows the infant to infer, by metaphor and analogy, forms of feeling "behind" the behavior. The infant detects whether or not the two separate minds are aligned to the same forms of feeling. Thus Stern's theory of intersubjectivity describes the origin of a symbolic mind....

Rizzolatti and Arbib (1998) suggest that mirror neurons provide an "action-recognition" mechanism: the actor's actions are reproduced in the premotor cortex of the observer. Wolf and colleagues (2001) suggest that through mirror neurons the observer has an enhanced capacity to recognize the intention of the actor. Pally (1999) puts it this way: I understand your intention by understanding what my own intention would be, if I were doing what you are doing....

Meltzoff holds that the infant maps the visually perceived behavior of the partner onto his own motor plans, Trevarthen proposes that the cerebral representations of the other is rooted in a motor image, and Stern conceptualizes the infant's capacity to "feel-what-has-been-perceived-in-the-other." The language of Meltzoff and Trevarthen comes very close to that of mirror neurons.

(pp. 51–53)

Research on Adult Attunement

Now we will examine how this base of attunement in infant research plays out in the adult therapeutic relationship. Daniel Siegel is a leading authority on interpersonal neurobiology. His book *The Developing Mind: Toward a Neurobiology of Interpersonal Experience* (Siegel, 1999) is the source of the following extracted paragraphs.

As this therapist and patient illustrate, engaging in direct communication is more than just understanding or even perceiving the signals—both verbal and nonverbal—sent between two people. For "full" emotional communication, one person needs to allow his state of mind to be influenced by that of the other (Trevarthen, 1993). In this example, the therapist's sensitivity to the patient's array of signals allows his own state to become aligned with that of the patient. The sense that his head is "about to burst," followed by the release of pressure, shows how the patient's shift from bewilderment to rage to sadness is experienced by the therapist. This shift in his own state may be a part of the internal process that makes him aware of the often subtle and rapid nonverbal signals sent in this direct form of emotional communication. The alignment of the therapist's state allows him to have an experience as close as possible to what the patient's subjective world is like at that moment. Sensitivity to signals allows for the therapist's internal response in his own state, which permits an awareness of his perceptions of the patient's experience. In addition to yielding important experiential information for the therapist, such an alignment permits a nonverbal form of communication to the patient that she is being "understood" in the deepest sense. Her state directly influences his; she is "feeling felt" by another person. This attunement of states forms the nonverbal basis of collaborative, contingent communication (Trevarthen, 1993). The capacity to achieve this attuned form of communication, sometimes called "affect attunement" (Stern, 1985; Haft and Slade, 1989), is dependent on an individual's sensitivity to signals. Parental sensitivity to signals is the essence of secure attachments (Ainsworth et al., 1978; de Wolff and van Ijzendoorn, 1997; Ward and Carlson, 1995) and can inform us about how two people's "being" with each other permits emotional communication and a sense of connection to be established at any age. In these transactions, the brain of one person and that of another are influencing each other in a form of "co-regulation" (Hofer, 1984)....

One essential message is that the developing mind uses the states of an attachment figure in order to help organize the functioning of its own states. The momentary alignment of states is dependent upon parental sensitivity to the child's signals and allows the mind of the child both to regulate itself in the moment and to develop regulatory capacities that can be utilized in the future (Schore, 1994; Oppenheim et al., 1997). The sensitivity to signals and attunement between child and parent, or between patient and therapist, involves the intermittent alignment of states of mind. As two individuals' states are brought into alignment, a form of what we can call "mental state resonance" can occur, in which each person's state both influences and is influenced by that of the other. There are moments in which people also need to be alone and not in alignment; an attuned other knows when to "back off" and stop the alignment process. Intimate relationships involve this circular dance of attuned communication, in which there are alternating moments of engaged alignment and distanced autonomy. At the root of such attunement is the capacity to read the signals (often nonverbal) that indicate the need for engagement or disengagement (Trevarthen, 1993).

As we shall see, states of mind involve various aspects of brain activity. The flow of energy and of information are both fundamental components of a state of mind. In this way, *attuned communication involves the resonance of energy and information.* For the nonverbal infant, this intimate, collaborative communication is without words. This need for nonverbal attunement persists throughout life. Within adult relationships of all sorts, words can come to dominate the form of information being shared, and this can lead to a different form of representational resonance. Such a verbal exchange may feel quite empty if it is devoid of the more primary aspects of each person's internal states (Stern, 1985). Infant attachment studies remind us of the crucial importance of nonverbal communication in all forms of human relationship.

(pp. 69–71)

Continuing in Siegel's book:

Peter Fonagy and colleagues have described this ability as a product of the adults' "reflective function," in which parents are able to reflect (using words) on the role of states of mind in influencing feelings, perceptions, intentions, beliefs, and behaviors (Fonagy et al., 1991; Fonagy and Target, 1997). For this reason, reflective function has been proposed to be at the heart of many secure attachments, especially when the parent has had a difficult early life. The nonverbal component of this reflective ability can be seen in the capacity for affect attunement as seen in these dyads, in which the emotional expression of each member of a pair is contingent with that of the other (Trevarthen, 1993). Attunement involves the alignment of states of mind in moments of engagement, during which affect is communicated with facial expression, vocalizations, body gestures, and eye contact. This attunement does not occur for every interaction (Bremner and Narayan, 1998, pp. 881–882). Rather, it is frequently present during intense moments of communication between infant and caregiver (Ochs and Capps, 1996; Coles, 1989).

   Healthy attunement therefore involves the parent's sensitivity to the child's signals and the collaborative, contingent communication that evokes what has been described earlier as a "resonance" between two people's states of mind: the mutual influence of each person's state on that of the other. Such attunement involves disengagement at moments when alignment is not called for and reengagement when both individuals are receptive to state-to-state connection. The states being aligned are indeed psychobiological states of brain activity (Field, 1985; Hofer, 1984; Trevarthen, 1993; Stern, 1985). Each individual becomes involved in a mutual co-regulation of resonating states (Hofer, 1994).

(p. 88)

Finally, the fourth book from which key paragraphs on attunement have been extracted is Pat Ogden's (with coauthors Kekuni Minton and Clare Pain) *Trauma and the Body: A Sensorimotor Approach to Psychotherapy* (Ogden, Minton, and Pain, 2006).

Working with traumatized individuals entails the overcoming of several major obstacles. One is that, although human contact and attunement are cardinal elements of physiological self-regulation, interpersonal trauma often results in a fear of intimacy. For many people the anticipation of closeness and attunement automatically evokes implicit memories of hurt, betrayal, and abandonment. As a result, feeling seen and understood—which helps most people feel calm and in control—may precipitate a reliving of the trauma in individuals who have been victimized in intimate relationships. Therefore, before trust can be established, it is important to help clients create a *physical* sense of control by working on the establishment of physical boundaries, exploring ways of regulating physiological arousal (using breath and body movement), and focusing on regaining a physical sense of being able to defend and protect themselves....

Another problem is that, neurobiologically speaking, the only part of the conscious brain that is capable of influencing emotional states (which are localized in the limbic system) is the medial prefrontal cortex, the part that is involved in introspection (i.e., attending to the internal state of the organism). Various neuroimaging studies reviewed in this book have shown decreased activation of the medial prefrontal cortex in individuals with PTSD (Lanius et al., 2002). This means that traumatized individuals, as a rule, have serious problems attending to their inner sensations and perceptions. When asked to focus on internal sensations, they tend to feel overwhelmed or deny having any. When they finally do pay attention to their inner world, they usually encounter a minefield of trauma-related perceptions, sensations, and emotions (Van der Kolk and Ducey, 1989). They often feel disgusted with themselves and usually have a very negative body image; as far as they are concerned, the less attention they pay to their bodies, the better. Yet one cannot learn to take care of oneself without being in touch with the demands and requirements of one's physical self.

Hence, Pat Ogden proposes that therapy is about learning to become a careful observer of the ebb and flow of internal experience, mindfully noticing whatever thoughts, feelings, body sensations, and impulses emerge. Traumatized individuals, first and foremost, need to learn that it is safe to have feelings and sensations. In this process it is critical for clients to become aware that bodily experience never remains static. Unlike at the moment of a trauma, when everything seems to freeze in time, physical sensations and emotions are in a constant state of flux.

(pp. xxiv–xxv)

Speaking of self-regulation:

The capacity to self-regulate is the foundation upon which a functional sense of self develops (Beebe and Lachmann, 1994; Schore, 1994; Stern, 1985). The sense of self is first and foremost a bodily sense, experienced not through language but through the sensations and movements of the body (Damasio, 1994, 1999; Janet, 1929; Krueger, 2002; Laplanche and Pontalis, 1998; Mahler and Furer, 1968; Stern, 1985). The primary sensations at the very beginning of life are physiological and tactile, and the primary form of communication immediately after birth between parent and newborn is through touch, with visual and auditory stimuli having a stronger role as times goes on (Krueger, 2002). The physical experience of the caregiver's gentle, attuned ministrations to the infant's signals pertaining to sensation, touch, movement, and physiological arousal, as well as to his or her sensitivities/vulnerabilities regarding sensory input and other physical needs (e.g., food, warmth, fluids) establishes the infant's initial sense of self and sense of his or her body (Gergely and Watson, 1996, 1999). Thus, "the close and careful attunement to all the sensory and motor contacts with the child forms an accurate and attuned body self in the child" (Krueger, 2002, p. 7). When this occurs, social engagement, secure attachment, and regulatory abilities are adaptively supported.

Early interpersonal trauma is not only a threat to physical and psychological integrity, but also a failure of the social engagement system. Moreover, if the perpetrator is a primary caregiver, it includes a failure of the attachment relationship, undermining the child's ability to recover and reorganize, to feel soothed or even safe again. The child's opportunity to effectively utilize social engagement for care and protection has been over ridden, and he or she experiences overwhelming arousal without the availability of attachment-mediated comfort or repair. Without adequate attunement and development of the social engagement system within a secure attachment relationship, "[c]hildren … are not able to create a sense of unity and continuity of the self across the past, present, and future, or in the relationship of the self with others. This impairment shows itself in the emotional instability, social dysfunction, poor response to stress, and cognitive disorganization and disorientation" (Siegel, 1999, pp. 119–120).

Understanding how self-regulatory capacities are formed through early attachment relationships is helpful to therapists, who also provide a similar relational context in which dysregulated clients can develop adaptive regulatory capacities (Beebe and Lachmann, 1994; Schore, 1994). In therapy, fostering clients' social engagement and regulatory abilities is a top priority.

Nonverbal cues are typically the first indicators of the client's experience of safety or danger in response to the therapeutic relationship, the environment, and internal cues (Lanyado, 2001). The therapist's attuned response to these nonverbal expressions is imperative in developing the client's social engagement system.

(pp. 42–43)

Ogden et al. define containment as a function of attunement:

Bion (1962) used the term *containment* to describe the primary caregiver's provision of a psychological environment that fosters the infant's self-regulating capacities. Winnicott's "holding environment" describes a similar concept that includes details about the type of physical care and environment that promote "the mental health of the infant" (1990, p. 49). By *containing* the child and providing a *holding environment,* the mother is able to hold the child both literally and in her mind in such a way that demonstrates her recognition of the child's physiological and affective states and also her ability to deal with them effectively. She can tolerate and "stay with" the child through his or her dysregulated states (Schore, 2003a).

Containment is communicated by the mother's holding and physical soothing of her infant's body with her touch and voice, which thereby modify the baby's physical sensations and motor activity (Brazelton, 1989). As the child develops, he or she acquires the capacity to experience security and comfort by means other than direct physical ministrations. Eye contact and words eventually "bridge the gap" between mother and child, and the child learns to calm down as the mother walks into his or her line of vision or is conjured in fantasy by the child as a comforting, calming presence.

(p. 44)

Then they discuss alignment and attunement:

One of the skills that enables mentalizing is the ability of the mother to perceive the child's world, identify with it, and align with it, while simultaneously realizing that the child is a separate person. Alignment—the empathic matching of one's own state to that of another Siegel (1999)—is a sensorimotor event that promotes social engagement communicated through prosody, voice tone and volume, touch, expression, pace, gestures, and so on. As the mother "gets closer to the child's state and then brings the child 'down' to a calmer state" (Siegel, 1999, pp. 280–281), through sensorimotor and emotional alignment, both mother and child experience a sense of calm and relaxation (Jaffe et al., 2001; Schore, 1994; Siegel, 1999; Stern, 1985).

In psychotherapy, attuned therapists need to provide *alignment* for clients, conveyed through voice tone, body language, and emotional "resonance" (Siegel, 1999), and *containment,* by helping them maintain arousal within the window of tolerance. As one client said, "I need to know that you won't let me go there [to the memories of the abuse]."

(pp. 44–45)

In a text section entitled "An Ever-Changing Body-to-Body Dialogue":

At the beginning of life, the newborn is dependent on its sensorimotor capacities (e.g., vocalizing, movement) to interact with the environment. However, social and emotional capacities quickly develop so that, by the end of the second month, the infant is able to engage in face-to-face interactions with the mother via intense and prolonged eye contact (Schore, 2003b). At this time, interactive play also begins, a highly arousing emotional and sensorimotor exchange in which the infant's rhythms and vocalizations are mirrored and elaborated by the mother (Schore, 2003b; Trevarthen, 1979). This body-to-body, brain-to-brain dialogue, described as "affect synchrony," is a give-and-take somatic exchange during which the mother facilitates the infant's information processing by "adjusting the mode, amount, variability, and timing of the onset and offset of stimulation to the infant's actual integrative capacities" (Schore, 2003b, p. 76). As the infant's affective body "language" is responded to in a pleasure-enhancing manner by an attuned caregiver, the positive experience of nonverbal communication fosters the development of the infant's sense of self and conditions his or her future relationship to somatic expression as a means of communication.

For this development to occur, caregivers must adapt to the infant's ongoing development: The "maturation of the nervous system, accompanied by increasing differentiation of skills, drives infants to reorganize their control systems. At each step, parents must also readjust, finding a new more appropriate way of reaching out" (Brazelton, 1989, p. 105). The caregiver's empathic discernment of the child's changing physical and emotional needs ensures a balance between an environment that is safe and secure and one that is sufficiently enriching to stimulate the child within his or her developmental capacity and to provide experiences of both enjoyment and mastery (Bradley, 2000; Emde, 1989).

(p. 45)

Research on Attention and Nature

According to Andrea Faber Taylor, an environmental psychologist and post-doctoral research associate at the University of Illinois, there are two kinds of attention. The first is the *directed attention* we call on for tasks that require focus, like driving or doing our taxes. Directed attention tends to be tiring, however, and fatigue affects our ability to make good decisions and control destructive impulses. The best way to restore directed attention is to give it a rest by shifting to the second type, *involuntary attention,* which we display when we watch the horizon while at the beach, stare at mountain tops, or meditate. Looking at nature is another activity that gives our directed attention a chance to recover. Some neurologists call these "focused attention" and "unfocused attention." The health of the brain and body depend on a balance of both kinds of attention. In terms of biodynamic craniosacral therapy, zone activity, especially attention in zone D, is a function of attunement that moves from focused to unfocused.

Roger Ulrich and his colleagues at Texas A&M University found that people who commuted along scenic roads recovered more quickly from stressful driving conditions than those who saw billboards, buildings, and parking lots. Ulrich also noted something he termed an *inoculation effect*: Drivers who had taken the scenic route responded more calmly to stressful situations later on. Ulrich also looked at patients recovering from gall bladder surgery. The patients who could see trees from their hospital beds needed fewer painkillers and had shorter hospital stays than those who looked out on brick walls.

So, with all our efforts to alleviate stress—from aerobics and yoga to anti-anxiety pills—maybe the key is as simple as gardening or taking a daily walk in the woods or on the beach. The lack of unfocused attention on nature is being linked to a host of health-care problems, including depression. These problems and symptoms are now being called nature deficit disorder. Even a little bit of green seems to make a big impact. Some studies suggest that a houseplant or even a picture of nature can convey similar benefits. Attunement with nature is a critical component of biodynamic practice.

Research on Zone B

In a finding that sheds new light on the neural mechanisms involved in social behavior, neuroscientists at the California Institute of Technology (Caltech) have pinpointed the brain structure responsible for our sense of personal space (Kennedy et al., 2009). The discovery, described in the August 30 issue of the journal *Nature Neuroscience,* could offer insight into autism and other disorders where social distance is a consideration.

The brain structure called the *amygdala*—a pair of almond-shaped regions located in the medial temporal lobes—was previously known to process strong negative emotions, such as anger and fear, and is considered the seat of emotion in the brain. However, it had never been linked rigorously to real-life human social interaction.

The Caltech experiment used what is known as the stop-distance technique. Briefly, the subject (one of twenty volunteers, representing a cross-section of age, ethnicity, education, and gender) stands a predetermined distance from an experimenter, then walks toward the experimenter and stops at the point where he or she feels most comfortable. The chin-to-chin distance between the subject and the experimenter is determined with a digital laser measurer.

Among the subjects, the average preferred distance was 0.64 meters—roughly 2 feet.

"Respecting someone's space is a critical aspect of human social interaction, and something we do automatically and effortlessly," Kennedy says. "These findings suggest that the amygdala, because it is necessary for the strong feelings of discomfort that help to repel people from one another, plays a central role in this process. They also help to expand our understanding of the role of the amygdala in real-world social interactions."

The Caltech colleagues then used a functional magnetic resonance imaging (fMRI) scanner to examine the activation of the amygdala in a separate group of healthy subjects who were told when an experimenter was either in close proximity or far away from them. When in the fMRI scanner, subjects could not see, feel, or hear the experimenter; nevertheless, their amygdalae lit up when they believed the experimenter to be close by. No activity was detected when subjects thought the experimenter was on the other side of the room.

"It was just the idea of another person being there, or not, that triggered the amygdala," Kennedy says. The study shows, he says, that "the amygdala is involved in regulating social distance, independent of the specific sensory cues that are typically present when someone is standing close, like sounds, sights, and smells."

The researchers believe that interpersonal distance is not something we consciously think about, although we become acutely aware when our space is violated. Kennedy recounts his own experience with having his personal space violated during a wedding: "I felt really uncomfortable, and almost fell over a chair while backing up to get some space." In biodynamic practice, the therapist must be acutely aware of this space, called zone B.

Across cultures, accepted interpersonal distances can vary dramatically, with individuals who live in cultures where space is at a premium (say, China or

Japan) seemingly tolerant of much closer distances than individuals in, say, the United States. (Meanwhile, our preferred personal distance can vary depending on our situation, making us far more willing to accept less space in a crowded subway car than we would be at the office.)

One explanation for this variation, Kennedy says, is that cultural preferences and experiences affect the brain over time and how it responds in particular situations. "If you're in a culture where standing close to someone is the norm, you'd learn that was acceptable and your personal space would vary accordingly," he says. "Even then, if you violate the accepted cultural distance, it will make people uncomfortable, and the amygdala will drive that feeling."

Part of biodynamic practice is to *deactivate* the amygdala and reduce the amount of fear in the client. This facilitates disengagement, ignition, and healing. This can occur by the practitioner's maintaining awareness of zone B, as suggested in Chapter 5. In my thirty-five years of clinical practice, I have seen the bodies of my clients become increasingly stressed. I have come to the conclusion that the human body was not designed for modern life. More than ever, now is the time to rethink, refeel, and refresh our relationship with natural world, which itself is the most vital aspect of the human body—nature.

CHAPTER 7

Interpersonal Neurobiology: Knowledge, Skills, and Abilities

This chapter covers the basic knowledge, skills, and abilities for the safe practice of biodynamic craniosacral therapy and the healthful development of the therapeutic relationship. It is based on the field of interpersonal neurobiology as discussed in this Volume Four and presented in table form, juxtaposing the knowledge about areas of work with the skills and abilities the practitioner needs to apply. The intent is make the individual principles more readily available to the practitioner to be applied in clinical practice.

Subsequent chapters will flesh out these skills in greater detail. The reader might well ask at the end of this chapter if it is necessary to know and practice each and every one of these skills. These skills take time to develop and gradually become second nature while with a client. I recommend picking one or two skills that are unfamiliar to the reader and getting to know their meaning and application. Then pick another one and so forth.

THERAPEUTIC RELATIONSHIP COMPETENCIES

Knowledge: Interpersonal neurobiology. Understand that cardiovascular and neurological self-regulation of the mind-body has two components: (1) internal self-regulation through conscious somatic awareness of the body from the inside, also called core regulation; and (2) self-regulation occurring socially in relationship through exteroceptive processing with the special senses of seeing, hearing, etc. (This is sometimes called the social nervous system.)	Skills and Abilities: Practitioner is responsible for building and maintaining a therapeutic container in which normal self-regulation can manifest in the practitioner and the client.

Knowledge: Understand that self-regulation is modulated by two pathways. One pathway is from the body and heart to the brain via sensation and feeling (bottom up) which is slower. It is simply energy and information to the brain. The second pathway is from the brain to the body via cognitive thinking (top down). This comes from a well-integrated prefrontal cortex. Biodynamic craniosacral therapy affects both pathways.	**Skills and Abilities:** Practitioner regularly senses the shape of his or her own body systemically as one whole continuum of fluid, bone, and membrane. This is three-dimensional fluid awareness. Practitioner maintains synchronization with Primary Respiration and stillness while orienting to the shape of his or her fluid body. This generates resonance with the client. Practitioner regularly scans his or her body from feet to head sensing the natural quiet under the skin. Practitioner intends to sense wholeness (indivisible connectedness) throughout the time of the session in self, space, and other. Practitioner periodically visualizes the client as one whole fluid continuum during a session.
Knowledge: Understand that self-regulation operates in three cotemporaneous neurological circuits: attunement, empathy, and intersubjectivity, which are all based on the quality of the practitioner's attention. There are five types of attention in biodynamic craniosacral therapy: focused, unfocused, deliberate, spontaneous, and resting.	**Skills and Abilities:** Practitioner maintains conscious awareness of mental and physical states while in relationship with the client. Practitioner regularly scans his or her own body from head to foot and inside to out through the zones in order to shift from focused attention to unfocused attention. Practitioner allows relaxation and openness to permeate his or her whole body out to the horizon and back at the tempo of Primary Respiration. Practitioner regularly breathes into the whole body from head to foot to synchronize with Primary Respiration. Practitioner rests his or her attention in the stillness when perceiving it three dimensionally in any of the zones.

Knowledge	Skills and Abilities
Knowledge: Understand the *first* neurological circuit, *attunement,* is the process in which the nervous systems of the practitioner and client maintain and build a therapeutic container based on safety and trust. Understand that attunement is based on the cycling of the practitioner's attention out through the zones and back in the tempo of Primary Respiration. At first this is a deliberate movement of attention and it gradually becomes spontaneous during a session.	**Skills and Abilities:** Practitioner becomes aware of the natural rhythm of attunement, which is how attention moves or toggles periodically between the body-mind of the practitioner and that of the client, out through the zones and back. Practitioner becomes aware of how attention naturally moves beyond the boundaries of the treatment room outside into nature and back rhythmically. Practitioner notices prolonged mental states that are disconnecting one's attention from the client or his or her body. Practitioner regularly moves attention back into his or her body gracefully and subtly. Practitioner uses conscious breathing to resynchronize with Primary Respiration in his or her fluid body.
Knowledge: Understand that under nonstressful conditions, the nervous systems of the client and the practitioner attune on average once per minute. (See Chapter 6.)	**Skills and Abilities:** Notice the speed or tempo of sensations, thoughts, and feelings in order to slow them down. Practitioner makes soft eye contact when appropriate with the client, especially before and after a session. Practitioner periodically visually scans the surface shape of the whole body of the client. Practitioner deliberately avoids fast tempos and tissue movement when encountering them in the client. Practitioner notices whether the client's breathing is synchronized with Primary Respiration. When stillness permeates the room, the practitioner takes time to notice it and rest in it.

Knowledge: Understand that the *second* neurological circuit, empathy, is generated in the brain and heart by *mirror neurons* in order to feel what the client is feeling (See Chapter 4 in Volume One.)	**Skills and Abilities:** Practitioner regularly focuses attention on the movement and activity of the heart and blood with the focused attention called interoceptive awareness or cardioception.
Understand that empathy is the foundation of compassion (caring and acting for the relief of pain and suffering of others).	Practitioner pays attention to the heartbeat pulsation spreading out to the hands and three dimensionally through his or her body.
Understand that the client and the practitioner coregulate each other's nervous systems and cardiovascular systems through mirroring and resonance, which generates emotional coherence (love, happiness, clarity, equanimity, kindness) and self-regulation.	Practitioner pays attention to his or her gut feelings such as tightening, cramping, queasiness, hunger, need for evacuation of the bowel or bladder, shifts in breathing, etc.
Understand that each person in the therapeutic relationship is affecting each other's nervous and cardiovascular systems equally whether with stress or with empathy.	Practitioner periodically might visualize the inside and outside of the client's body as a three-dimensional undifferentiated fluid shape or a differentiated anatomical shape.
Understand that the practitioner's empathy develops a felt sense in the client of being nurtured and loved.	Practitioner periodically maintains attention on his or her trunk, abdomen, and diaphragm for any sensations and feelings to facilitate empathy.
Understand that empathy and compassion are built through the conscious somatic awareness of the practitioner.	Practitioner notices sensations of heat and warmth and allows them to permeate the body systemically.
Understand that compassion is the foundation of moral development. Biodynamic craniosacral therapy facilitates moral development.	Practitioner periodically smiles as a type of nonverbal dialogue between practitioner and client.
	Practitioner regularly senses the motion of the blood under his or her skin.
	Practitioner actively senses the inside of his or her hands as continuous or connected with the heart.

Knowledge: Nurturing physical touch when coupled with empathy stimulates the release of the hormone oxytocin, associated with the felt sense of love in both the practitioner and the client.	**Skills and Abilities:** Practitioner periodically contemplates the flow of Primary Respiration as loving kindness flowing from the heart through the hands while in contact with the client.
	Practitioner contemplates the client's history sensing Primary Respiration moving from his or her heart to the client and back while doing an intake or even while in contact with the client.
	Whenever appropriate, the practitioner might imagine being a mother or father holding and feeding a newborn baby when in contact with the client. The reverse is also true in that the client could be the practitioner's mother, and the practitioner the client's child.
	Practitioner employs buoyant touch during a session.
	Practitioner regularly senses the back of the hands connected to the back of his or her body.

Knowledge: Understand that clients hold stress, trauma, and shock in their fluid body and soma, which are capable of being sensed by the practitioner before, during, and after a session through neurological resonance with the client.	**Skills and Abilities:** Practitioner periodically attends to thoughts, feelings, emotions, and sensations while in contact with the client and acknowledges them by postural shifting, removing one's hands from the client, or moving one's attention through the zones and resting in stillness.
	Practitioner observes signs of the client's autonomic nervous system seeking homeostasis such as skin color tone, breathing, shaking or trembling, eyes glazing, etc.
	Practitioner modulates contact with the client slowly while the autonomic nervous system is active. (This is especially relevant in the first three sessions with a client.)
	Practitioner acknowledges strong sensations in his or her body with conscious breathing and mental clearing.
	Practitioner brackets or saves personal feelings and emotions that persist in a session for reflection after the client has left the office.
	Practitioner seeks supervision if thoughts, feelings, and emotions that come up in a client session trigger personal history or a personal emotional process.
	Practitioner consciously notices a range of feelings from irritability all the way to feelings of sexual intimacy toward the client when it occurs.
	Practitioner maintains clear, responsible, and conscious boundaries with clients.
Knowledge: Understand that the *third* neurological circuit, intersubjectivity, is a part of the nervous systems of the client and practitioner remaining oriented to present time rather than the past or future.	**Skills and Abilities:** Practitioner breathes into thoughts of the past and future to release them.
	Practitioner synchronizes his or her breathing with Primary Respiration frequently during a session.
	Practitioner is willing to feel awkward or make an occasional mistake during a session.

Knowledge: Understand that clear verbal communication is an important boundary and facilitates successful health outcomes.	Skills and Abilities: Practitioner actively listens to the client without distracting personal thoughts.
	Practitioner actively acknowledges the client as they speak through soft eye contact, head nodding, sounds of recognition, and/or words of recognition.
	Practitioner verbally reflects the client's story back to him or her, either in segments or in total as time permits. Listen to the client as if trying to memorize each word he or she is saying.
	Practitioner is curious, but not obtrusive, if something in the client's story seems to be missing.
	Practitioner avoids provoking client's emotions through verbal or manual techniques.

Tips for Dealing with Emotional Release

The following list is reprinted with permission from *The Psychology of the Body* by Elliot Greene and Barbara Goodrich-Dunn (2004, p. 124).

- Be present!
- You do not need to "do" anything.
- Feelings are not harmful.
- Keep breathing; remain centered and grounded (yourself).
- Encourage the client to keep breathing.
- Facilitate grounding (by the client).
- Allow time for quiet, if needed.
- Allow time for talk, and to ask questions, if needed.
- Use reflective listening when appropriate.
- Be supportive, nonjudgmental, and accepting.
- Maintain a safe space for the client.
- Respect what has happened; remember this may be a very important event in the client's life.
- Refrain from giving advice.
- Own your feelings; i.e., honestly acknowledge and take responsibility for how you are feeling (to yourself).

- Refrain from withdrawal, judgment, and using psychotherapeutic methods.
- In the long term, increase self-awareness and work to become more comfortable with the feelings with which you are not comfortable.

Differentiating between Handling and Processing Psychological Material

The massage therapist (or craniosacral therapist) is *not* trained to *process* psychological material. This work falls within the domain of psychotherapy and requires a graduate degree and professional licensing. Greene and Goodrich-Dunn (2004, p. 71) list activities that are more the role of a psychotherapist rather than a craniosacral therapist, and involve *processing;* this list is also reprinted with permission.

- Eliciting or encouraging the client to give more information
- Encouraging stronger emotional release
- Suggesting what the emotional material might be related to
- Focusing on emotional problems
- Interpreting either verbal information or emotional expression
- Talking about transference issues
- Deepening transference by encouraging exploration of whom the therapist represents and how the client feels about that person

The massage therapist (or craniosacral therapist) may *handle* psychological material. Handling psychological material involves the following:

- Acknowledging the presence of psychological material when it appears
- Using active listening and reflection
- Providing nonjudgmental support
- Being present and centered
- Creating a safe environment
- Helping the client ground him- or herself through the body
- Making an appropriate referral if needed

Knowledge, or knowing something, can be differentiated from the skills and abilities necessary for handling or processing the material being dealt with in a practitioner–client interaction.

The lists below juxtapose the knowledge against the skills and abilities, with regard to areas commonly dealt with by craniosacral therapists.

DEALING WITH PAST SHOCK EXPERIENCES

Knowledge: Understand that body language, some postures, and certain body shapes and forms are visible expressions of early psychological history coupled to chronic stress, traumatization, and experiences of shock in the past.	**Skills and Abilities:** Practitioner observes the client's posture and movement as an active shaping process from early embryonic development.
Understand that such chronic shape changes imprinted on the body are referred to as *character structure*. Character structure is held in place by *character armoring*. Both create a psychosomatic body and generate a sense of fragmentation or lack of wholeness.	Practitioner notices that when the client's body does not relax or become buoyant, it may be armored and held by unconscious prenatal experience that needs to be normalized with Primary Respiration.
Understand in such cases, that structural and functional considerations are secondary to the psychological component. The psychological component is secondary to the biodynamic component of Primary Respiration breathing the whole fluid body.	Practitioner does not pathologize the client consciously (or unconsciously). Rather, the practitioner normalizes his or her observations and sees the client as whole.
	Practitioner occasionally asks the client to breathe into his or her hands.
Understand that character structure and armoring are rooted in the normal prenatal development of an embryo and fetus.	Practitioner moves on to another area of the client's body if one area is unresponsive to Primary Respiration or stillness.
	Practitioner seeks specialized training to work with body psychotherapy and trauma resolution. It is not combined with biodynamic craniosacral therapy in one session but can be adjunctive in some cases.

DEALING WITH ILLNESS

Knowledge: Understand that disease and illness have numerous focal points of origin from pre-conception through the life span.	**Skills and Abilities:** Practitioner avoids interpretation of the client's story.
	Practitioner avoids judgment of the client's story.
	Practitioner is willing to *not* know the source or cause of a client's pain and suffering.
	Practitioner allows space and builds a container of tolerance for the amazing diversity of backgrounds (race, color, creed, etc.) that each client is.
	Practitioner develops patience.
	Practitioner develops stillness.
	Practitioner maintains focus on his or her personal development of self-regulation skills.
	Practitioner is thoroughly familiar and operates with a rigorous code of ethics.

CHAPTER 8

Disengagement and Self-Regulation in Biodynamic Practice

I want to discuss the new science of interpersonal neurobiology (IPNB), specifically the autonomic nervous system and biodynamic practice. IPNB describes the way in which the nervous and vascular systems of two people in relationship merge together. It is based on the discovery of mirror neurons in the brain and heart. This means that all humans have the capacity to mirror the feelings of another person. In other words, everyone has the innate capacity to experience the emotions of another person. This is called empathy and can be enhanced for therapeutic value and healing with a specific type of sensory awareness.

To begin a discussion of sensory awareness, I will start with the autonomic nervous system and how it functions. Disengagement is a term in biodynamic craniosacral therapy that refers to the normalization of tone in the autonomic nervous system (ANS) and then the initiation of a biodynamic therapeutic process. The autonomic nervous system is described as having two parts, the sympathetic nervous system (SNS) and the parasympathetic nervous system (PNS). Fight-flight and hyperarousal states (SNS) as well as immobile-freezing states (PNS) disengage and are contained within a window of normal tolerance of the daily ups and downs of stress such as the heart rate, which is coregulated by the ANS. Normalization of high and low ANS tone must occur as a function of the therapeutic relationship when touch is involved. When the tone in the autonomic nervous system normalizes, Primary Respiration (a slow tempo) can begin to manifest more of its potency in the client's therapeutic process. I teach a five-step process regarding the observation and contact that the practitioner has with the client regarding both of their ANSs. The reader can review Chapter 27 in Volume Three for a complete explanation of the five-step process. This chapter will briefly describe activation, stabilization, disengagement, self-regulation, and empathy as the core of IPNB.

The first step is to understand that the contemporary client typically goes through many phases of ANS activation and settling during the day. This means that the autonomic nervous system cycles between an alarm state and/or a fight-flight state (sympathetic states—SNS), followed by a phase of withdrawing, immobility or freezing states (parasympathetic states—PNS) outside the normal tolerance levels. This entire cycling phenomenon has been well documented in the trauma resolution research that I discussed in Volume Two. The point is whether or not the client can escape abnormal cycling (hyperarousal-hypoarousal states) by entering a phase of *relaxation* followed by longer periods of *stabilization* within a window of normal tolerance. Stabilization then leads to *self-regulation.* Self-regulation refers to the ability of the prefrontal cortex of the brain to be aware and calm no matter what is happening in or out of the body. In this chapter, it is called "the central stillness." The prefrontal cortex of the brain is described as the executive control center of the brain for down-regulating the ANS, as I discussed at length in Volume One.

Clinically, the first several sessions of biodynamic craniosacral therapy with a new client focus on observing how the client cycles in the ANS. Does the client have an ANS capable of self-regulation and stabilization by itself? ANS cycling without self-regulation and stabilization is a form of volatile combustion. Combustion overcharges the client's nervous system and body resulting in imbalances at all levels of structure and function. The client lives a lot of his or her life outside the window of normal tolerance for the ANS. Symptoms of imbalance may include elevated heart rate (heart disease), muscle pain (chronic low back pain), insomnia, strong emotional swings, depression, and anxiety, to name a few possibilities among many.

Another clinical point here is that touch itself can also be activating for the client. This is due to a part of the brain, the insular cortex, that reads the context of the touch. The insular cortex determines whether the touch is loving or stressful. This part of the brain is especially active in infants who spend the majority of their time in the first year after birth being held by a caregiver. Since there may be challenges to experiencing safety from the caregiver at this time of life in at least half the population, the insular cortex is not able to discern the context of loving touch and allow the whole body a love-relaxation response. Thus, therapeutic touch may in fact be activating for the adult client's ANS from this preverbal implicit memory. Consequently, the loving touch may be reinforcing a fight-flight tendency or immobility without calming either the fight-flight or the immobility. The client has no conscious recall of not being safe as an infant, yet the implicit memory remains in the adult brain and body and manifests as physical or behavioral symptoms.

This brings us to the second step of stabilization regarding the ANS. For a client to advance clinically, I strongly believe that the volatile combustion of the autonomic nervous system must be able to achieve stability by itself or with the help of a trained trauma resolution specialist or health care practitioner. Stabilization is an important stage to achieve in the biodynamic healing process. Frequently, stabilization takes time to have a noticeable effect on the day-to-day activity of a client at a conscious level. Follow-up sessions in biodynamic practice help stabilize, relax, and normalize the ANS. Such stability is needed to reprogram the prefrontal cortex to take control.

Sometimes, stabilization cannot occur without proper medication, dietary changes, and/or lifestyle changes. These are significant therapeutic pieces that require a good referral base to other health care practitioners who have such expertise. However, I also believe and have observed clinically that a client can become stable through the self-regulation skills of a biodynamic practitioner. This is a core principle in the field of interpersonal neurobiology. Conscious awareness of one's heartbeat, breathing, and the sensory awareness of the whole of the body are some of the important skills necessary for the biodynamic practitioner. Thus, I have frequently said in classes that the practitioner spends the majority of a therapeutic session perceiving his or her own body and self-regulating thoughts, feelings, and emotions as they arise in the body and mind. These skills go beyond the treatment room and become a way of life.

The third step regarding the autonomic nervous system and its biodynamic therapeutic process is disengagement. Disengagement specifically means that states of hyperarousal (fight-flight) and hypoarousal (withdrawal) in the client's ANS have dissipated, at least temporarily. When you step on the clutch and get the car out of gear, it simply begins to idle without surging and lurching forward and backward. Disengagement is an indication that the client's autonomic nervous system has begun to stabilize by becoming still or idle, and is beginning to regain its capacity to self-regulate and recalibrate the whole nervous and cardiovascular systems toward normal. Disengagement allows the fluid body to begin to normalize and be influenced by the slow tempo of Primary Respiration. (The term *fluid body* is defined and discussed in depth in Volumes One through Three.) In short, the fluid body is the original body in our embryonic beginnings. It existed prior to a brain and heart and still functions in the adult body as a holistic system. Disengagement facilitates the recalibration of the heart, brain, and blood. Furthermore, the volatile combustion of the ANS can be transformed into ignition and a deeper level of healing, as discussed in the next chapter. I have also written about ignition in all three of my previous volumes.

Some teachers refer to an event immediately following disengagement as a *neutral* or the *holistic shift* in which Primary Respiration is free to initiate its therapeutic process in the client's body for renewal and repair. Disengagement is an indication that the emphasis of Primary Respiration has shifted from maintaining the health of the body to repairing the wholeness of the fluid body with the help of the heart and blood. Dr. William Garner Sutherland sensed this event of disengagement and neutral as the perception of "idling" in the client's body. In biodynamic practice, Dr. Rollin Becker said that this is the *actual beginning* of the therapeutic process. Since disengagement is also associated with stillness and slowness, many practitioners mistake disengagement as the *end point* of a therapeutic process. This is incorrect discernment. It is the actual beginning of the biodynamic therapeutic process.

At a physiological level, disengagement means that the sympathetic and parasympathetic branches of the ANS have regained a measure of their reciprocal function for self-correction. This means that the sympathetic and parasympathetic branches of the ANS have recoupled back to their normal functioning of achieving equilibrium after a change process. Some authors call this process of achieving equilibrium *homeostasis* and others call it *allostasis* (McEwen, 2002). The ANS can avoid getting stuck in the sympathetic highs of hyperarousal and fight-flight and the parasympathetic lows of withdrawing and freezing. Of course, this beneficial recoupling and rebalancing is likely to be sensed as a seismic event in the client's body by a practitioner and even by some clients in themselves. However, remember, it is the beginning and not the end of the biodynamic therapeutic process. Frequently a client will report experiences of buoyancy using metaphors of the ocean, such as waves or currents, or feel very tired and go home and sleep for twelve hours. This is a clear indication of the therapeutic shift from the ANS to the wholeness of fluid body. It is a hallmark of disengagement.

Disengagement is facilitated by the self-regulation skills of the practitioner. This is not exactly a linear process since the practitioner will be using his or her self-regulation skills from the beginning of the session. After disengagement occurs, self-regulation skills can deepen into a more clear awareness of Primary Respiration and stillness for longer periods of time. The client's whole body is recalibrating between the fluid body, heart-blood, and nervous system. There are numerous self-regulation skills that the practitioner uses consciously, even with hands on the client. Some of these skills include:

- Performing regular body scans in one's body to maintain a sense of wholeness and three dimensionality

- Interoception, or paying attention to one's heartbeat and movement of the blood from the core of the body to the periphery and back

- Maintaining contact with the ebb and flow of warmth and heat in the body, especially when in contact with a client

- Moving attention slowly through the zones of perception that include the practitioner's body, the office space, and the world of nature outside

- Conscious breathing

Whatever appropriate skill the practitioner uses to become more consciously aware of the present moment is valuable and builds empathy.

These self-regulation skills are important aspects of the new science of IPNB. Now we are back to the opening paragraph of this chapter. One of the very important IPNB skills for the practitioner to cultivate is the ability to access a central stillness in one's mind and body. Daniel Siegel calls this "mindsight" (Siegel, 2010). A Buddhist might call this mindfulness. I have also heard it called the silent witness or witness consciousness. Nonetheless, these metaphors speak to an intrinsic capacity that everybody has to be inwardly or mentally quiet. This includes a deeper stillness that contains a faculty of awareness that can observe sensations, feelings, emotions, and thoughts that constantly stream through the body-mind with a sense of equanimity. Such awareness and self-regulation skills light up the prefrontal cortex in brain research studies. This is covered in detail in Volume One.

As Jon Kabat-Zinn says in his book *Coming to Our Senses* (2005, p. 88), "awareness of fear is not afraid …, awareness of depression is not depressed …, awareness of your bad habits is not a slave to those bad habits." This simple awareness of peace and equanimity is embedded in our bodily life everywhere, not just in the prefrontal cortex. The fluid body, the heart, and blood are also organs of perception for stillness and equanimity. This is a deeper shift in one's relationship with any experience that gives more freedom and power to change the experience. Even not knowing is a kind of knowing when embraced in awareness.

Interpersonal neurobiology has its basis in understanding the nine functions of the prefrontal cortex. These functions are:

- Bodily regulation

- Attuned communication

- Emotional balance

- Response flexibility

- Fear modulation

- Empathy

- Insight

- Moral awareness

- Intuition

This list and commentary on it can be found in Daniel Siegel's book *Mindsight: The New Science of Personal Transformation* (2010). These functions are built, maintained, and repaired through the practitioner's skills mentioned above and many other skills as well. I believe that the most important skill is being able to consciously rest in the central stillness in the middle of mind, heart, and fluid body. This builds the power of reflection and equanimity and supports all nine functions listed above. This deepens empathy into compassionate action. It overcomes many difficult emotions, especially shame. It minimizes the projection and transference process psychologically between people, especially in the therapeutic relationship. It is the essence of forgiveness. It is from this central stillness that the practitioner learns to be open, to observe clearly, and to be objective, not only with oneself, but also in all human relationships. This type of reflection gives power to the repair and reconnection necessary in so many human relationships and that includes the client-therapist relationship. Such reflection supports disengagement of the autonomic nervous system and the biodynamic therapeutic process under the control of Primary Respiration. It further generates greater discernment and correct knowing, not only in one's own mind and body, but also in the client's mind and body through the resonance of brain to brain and heart to heart.

The ability to rest in the central stillness of the body, heart, and mind actively shapes the structure and function of the brain. By maintaining a conscious perception of the three-dimensional shape of the body, spending more time with interoceptive awareness or attention on the heart and breathing, the brains of both the practitioner and client will be able to reshape and reinhabit more fully the nine prefrontal functions mentioned above. According to Siegel (1999), mental activity and brain firing (function) are a two-way street. Genes, chance, and experience shape the brain from inside out and outside in. This is well known in the research literature (Meaney, 2010).

It is now said that pre-conception experience from our great grandparents shapes the brain in terms of genetic patterns. The eggs and sperm of our ancestors can be imprinted with stress that may manifest as disease in later generations. This comes from the field of epigenesis. Emotions are really just energy and information. The human mind via the prefrontal cortex and heart is a relational and embodied process that regulates the two forms of mental experience, energy, and information. Energy and information keep flowing through the body and brain. The body is a moving process of formation. One can step into the flow of energy and information and change it whether that is the movement of thoughts, emotions, or the blood and heart. Minds have unique abilities to shape the flow through conscious attention to the central stillness and the slowness of Primary

Respiration. Conscious awareness of the body and its core viscera changes brain structure and function, especially toward empathy.

The most fundamental principle of interpersonal neurobiology is that conscious attention and awareness periodically oriented to the central stillness permit a person to direct the flow of energy and information toward integration and normalization of life experience. Mindful awareness or mindsight, again as Siegel calls it, is a combination of insight and empathy. The biggest revolution in the neurological sciences since the discovery of the DNA-RNA complex has been the discovery of mirror neurons. Mirror neurons reflect what is being observed in another person and generate a field of energy and information in the brain that closely resembles what the other person is feeling. This neurological field is then brought down into the whole physical body of the observer. Thus, each person can sense the feelings of another person in his or her body. Other researchers have argued that mirror neurons can also be found in the heart and thus influence the way the heart coregulates the flow of information and energy in the brain. IPNB is the new science of empathy and compassion.

The circuits of mirror neurons, whether limited to the brain or expanded to include their heart–brain connection, create resonance circuits. Resonance circuits generate much deeper physiological synchronization between two people, especially between a practitioner and a client. In other words, empathy builds empathy, which leads to a deeper and stronger sense of compassionate action, which ultimately leads to a deeper sense of altruistic love and kindness, not just for a client, but also for everyone. This is the arc of altruism that starts with empathy. Deep healing can occur when the client feels *felt* by the therapist and likewise the therapist feels *felt* by the client. This is empathy and compassion at work and it is a natural and normal function of the mind and body.

The awareness of another person's state of mind and body depends on how well a practitioner knows his or her own mind and body. It is clear now from the research that people who are more aware of their bodies are more empathetic. More empathy leads to less disruption of the autonomic nervous system outside the normal window of tolerance. It is important, however, to differentiate mirroring from resonance. Mirroring has a tendency to be confusing. Frequently, I hear students report being merged with a client and losing objectivity. Resonance requires that the practitioner knows who he or she is while at the same time being in contact with another person, especially with the hands. Practitioners allow their internal states to be influenced by the client but not to become identical with those states in the other person. This is done by the practitioner opening to his or her own body, heart movement, belly sensation, breathing, and, above all, resting in the central stillness. It is a lifelong learning process and something not mastered in a short period of time.

This chapter started with a discussion of the ANS and its need for stability and disengagement. The description of these important principles of interpersonal neurobiology are focused once again on the practitioner's ability to self-regulate and become more conscious of his or her body. Consciousness of the body includes those elements discussed above. Consciousness of the body is not limited to these skills, but by orienting to the central stillness, insight arises that guides the practitioner into a much deeper level of practice and sensibility of a two-person biology. The therapeutic relationship by its nature is very fluid and buoyant.

To review, the therapeutic process regarding disengagement of the ANS goes through five phases.:

- First, observing the client's autonomic activation

- Second, a phase of autonomic stabilization

- Third, the biodynamic phase of disengagement, in which Primary Respiration is able to manifest its known potency

- Fourth, the self-regulation skills of the practitioner, applied for resonance with the client

- Fifth, the practitioner deepening into empathy and therapeutic insight that arises from empathy, and leading to compassionate action

To accomplish the skillful disengagement of a client's autonomic nervous system, the practitioner must understand and practice these interpersonal neurobiology principles, occasionally sample a good bottle of wine, and especially have a sense of humor about one's place in the universe.

Of the many principles of interpersonal neurobiology, the most important in my clinical experience is the ability of the practitioner to consciously rest in the central stillness. This central stillness lives in the body and its perception expands out to the horizon and back, generating a living connection to our wholeness with all things. This is followed closely by consciously enhancing empathy and compassion through sensing one's heart and blood movement. This is one of the deepest ways to allow the ANS to disengage, regulate, and balance itself in one's self and other. When the practitioner has firsthand experience of his or her autonomic nervous system disengaging, through resonance, the client is also shown the way to disengage his or her ANS. This is self-regulation through resonance. Maybe some old karmic and behavioral habits are immune to any substantial change unless the person is open or ready for change. This, however, opens the door for Primary Respiration to become a function of empathy in the practitioner. Empathy flows in all directions and biodynamic practice becomes a protocol for compassion and loving kindness.

Thank you to my brother Brian Shea, Sara Dochterman, and my wife Cathy for their editing and shaping of the ideas in this chapter.

CHAPTER 9

Ignition

Judging by what I have learned about men and women, I am convinced that far more idealistic aspiration exists than is ever evident. Just as the rivers we see are much less numerous than the underground streams, so the idealism that is visible is minor compared to what men and women carry in their hearts, unreleased or scarcely released. Mankind is waiting and longing for those who can accomplish the task of untying what is knotted and bringing the underground waters to the surface.

(Albert Schweitzer)

Sometimes the term *ignition* is confusing. This is because it is used to describe a discrete process within Primary Respiration, one phase in that process, and the end of the five-step biodynamic process as I describe it. The term is used loosely to describe other perceptions during biodynamic practice as well. I would like to clarify some of the confusion by offering simple definitions and alternatives to the perceptual process called ignition. To begin, I define ignition as the innate ability to create, repair, and maintain the balance of life forces in the body, mind, and natural world. It is the spontaneous pulse of transformation during important transitions in a person's life, such as birth and death, marriage and divorce, and so forth. It provides meaning to support differentiated wholeness during the life span. This to me is the big picture with ignition in biodynamic practice. Now let's look at some different but related layers of meaning for ignition.

In biodynamic craniosacral therapy, the term ignition refers to a five-phase process within the cycles of Primary Respiration and is used as an adjective within that five-phase process, such as when it changes phases between coming in and going out. I also use the term as the final stage of the biodynamic process of orienting, synchronizing, attuning, disengaging, and igniting. Chapter 27 in Volume Three includes an overview of these stages. When I refer to ignition this way, I mean it to refer to the five phases of ignition in Primary Respiration, which I will cover below.

Ignition is also used to describe such phenomena in nature as a sunrise or a tsunami, and to the smallest events in a person's body, such as a deep breath. It can be painful or joyous or anything in between. Ignition carries the potential for transformation, and this depends on the perception of the practitioner. In all of these usages, the common element is the notion of transition from one state to another, whether cognitively or physically.

Ignition is the engine, the deep pulse so to speak, of the therapeutic processes under the direction of the rhythmic balanced interchange of Primary Respiration and Dynamic Stillness. It can be split into five parts, as mentioned, but it is clearly the dynamo of Primary Respiration. I will go into more detail on the biodynamic therapeutic processes in Chapter 21. Ignition is thus a category of discrete perception in the ongoing therapeutic relationship. Such perception can be localized to the client and practitioner or become nonlocal through the zones and life in general. Being able to recognize its sensibilities in both biodynamic practice and life in general leads to deeper and more meaningful healing. This is because ignition is a cause for the integration of life experience into a more differentiated living wholeness. As with acupuncture, ignition is the pulse of the deeper energy systems of the fluid body and nature. It is the type of pulse, however, that can be read by the practitioner as it spontaneously appears in any of the zones of perception and gradually in life.

Ignition infers the active presence of a fulcrum or functional midline that is capable of expanding out through the zones, which I will discuss below. The fulcrum or midline *is the stillness* and is constantly dancing together with Primary Respiration as one thing. In other words, Primary Respiration and stillness are one thing. Our nervous system and senses make it two things. The fulcrum or midline and stillness are also one thing. Primary Respiration, stillness, and the fulcrum or midline are thus simply one thing, a living continuum of wholeness that is indivisible. Avoid the confusion of treating them as separate whenever possible.

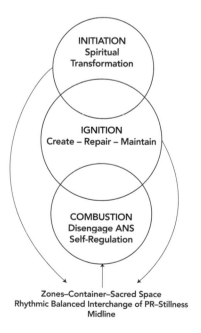

BIODYNAMICS OF IGNITION

INITIATION
Spiritual
Transformation

IGNITION
Create – Repair – Maintain

COMBUSTION
Disengage ANS
Self-Regulation

Zones–Container–Sacred Space
Rhythmic Balanced Interchange of PR–Stillness
Midline

Figure 9.1. The continuum of ignition

Zones

The pulse of ignition is perceived as discrete phenomena such as the transition from one phase of Primary Respiration to its other phase. It is capable of initiating a healing or therapeutic process in one or all of the zones of perception (see Chapter 5), but not always. Only the skill and practice of the practitioner can discriminate between the value of ignition events in any of the zones. The zones denote *boundaries of awareness* of three-dimensional space. They are artificial but useful distinctions in therapeutic practice, because they provide the container for the healing process. The zones in biodynamic practice are generally differentiated as:

- Zone A, the body bounded by the skin
- Zone B, the space around the body out to about twenty inches off the skin, sometimes referred to as the boundary of the fluid body
- Zone C, the space bounded by the walls, ceiling, and floor
- Zone D, the natural world outside the window out to the horizon

The client has the same zones that are intermingling with the practitioner's. The zones are metaphors or images of three-dimensional space and full of clinical relevance for the practitioner. This means that, whether the image or metaphor takes the form of a beam of sunlight coming through the window of the office, thunder and lightning, bird song coming from the trees, a sudden deep stillness in the office, an increase in the practitioner's heart rate, or a client's spontaneous deep inhalation, any and all are possibly ignition related. Gradually, the boundaries between the zones disappear in clinical practice and they become merged with the wholeness.

Phases

Ignition has previously been defined in my books as a sequence of perceptual processes or phases occurring as a continuum through both phases of Primary Respiration. There is the practitioner's perception of Primary Respiration and then a sublevel or layer of perception related to ignition. In other words, Primary Respiration has numerous levels to it and ignition is simply one of those levels. Think of these different phases as pulses that are either weak or strong. These five perceptual events are described below.

- The *spark* (of the Breath of Life, according to Dr. Sutherland) occurs briefly at the beginning of Primary Respiration going out to the horizon from one of its fulcrums (umbilicus, heart, and third ventricle) in the fluid body. If a practitioner thinks and senses reciprocally then when Primary Respiration is returning from the horizon in zone D it is possible that it is not just returning from his or her vantage point but rather an intelligence is breathing Primary Respiration to us as a form of expansion. Many students have reported such a perception. I feel that the term spark is more accurate for many of the experiences that practitioners report in a session.

- *Ignition,* or *combustion,* which I prefer, is a term derived from automobile terminology and used by Dr. Sutherland to indicate how the turning of the key causes a spark that turns on the whole engine in a car. In this case the combustion of ignition initiates a potent expression of Primary Respiration. I like the term combustion. After the spark, there is a spontaneous combustion of life force in the midline of the body. In this case combustion is contained in the midline and is thus available for permeation of the potencies of Primary Respiration. When combustion is uncontained, the autonomic nervous system does not function optimally.

- In *permeation,* Primary Respiration and its potency spread and move through the fluid body in a three-dimensional spatial (positional) relationship to one or all of the three embryonic fulcrums. (This will be discussed at length in the chapters on the hand positions.)

- The *augmentation* phase occurs at the end of Primary Respiration coming in from the horizon to one of its fulcrums (Primary Respiration naturally and normally enhances itself by its interchange with Dynamic Stillness or by being in contact with the practitioner who is aware of such phenomena). I like to think of this phase as a type of refueling, in which Primary Respiration is given added fuel to initiate the change of phase and initiating spark of combustion.

- In the *disengagement* phase the central and autonomic nervous systems of the client achieve a point of stability, with automatic shifting of strains in the fluid body toward normal and for Primary Respiration to initiate a deeper level of self-correction in the fluid body and beyond. (This was discussed in detail in the preceding chapter.)

It is important to remember that these events are not always localized inside the body of the practitioner and/or the client. They have continuity through all the zones in both the practitioner and the client. In other words, a spark can occur in zone D, augmentation can occur in zone C, and so forth. The therapeutic relevance of such phenomena is very contextual and depends on both the client's and the practitioner's experience.

Fulcrum

Ignition as a process occurs in relationship to the original four embryonic fulcrums that precede the structural midline. These four fulcrums are related to the four spheres of fluid that the embryo forms beginning at the second week postfertilization. They are the umbilicus (yolk sac), third ventricle (amniotic sac), the heart (chorion sac), and the allantois (bladder).

Clinically, the practitioner observes these fulcrums and whether they are balanced to one another. Since all fulcrums automatically shift in relationship to each other, the practitioner simply uses the skills detailed in Chapters 15–21 to balance these four critical fulcrums in biodynamic practice. All three fulcrums express the rhythmic balanced interchange of Primary Respiration and Dynamic Stillness. All structure in the human body is oriented to this functional interchange as a living, breathing movement in the embryonic fulcrums. One teacher calls these four fulcrums the horizontal midlines. This is because they are relational midlines. The umbilicus extends to the uterus via the placenta. The heart extends to the heart of the mother in utero and all other hearts after birth. The third ventricle extends to the brain of the mother and subsequently all other brains after birth. The allantois looks like a tiny bladder and induces the umbilical vein and artery to form from the placenta before it becomes the anterior bladder much later in development.

Midline

The midline itself is described in a wide variety of ways in the osteopathic and craniosacral therapy communities. It has many different aspects structurally, functionally, and archetypally (spiritually), which I have described in various writings of mine (see all of my previous volumes). Consequently, a practitioner can stay quite busy or confused trying to sort out all of these meanings in clinical practice. Practically, I am focusing on what I feel is the most important function of the midline unique to all of them in this chapter: the practitioner's perception of the interchange of Primary Respiration and Dynamic Stillness.

Sensing the fulcrums and the midline as this interchange is first a perceptual experience and the practitioner must be guided by her body. This is the deepest function and experience of the fulcrums and midline. In other words, the specific location of the fulcrums and the midline are quite variable. They can expand to fill the body and the zones and just be one whole living dynamic rather than a location or structure. They can automatically shift from inside the body to outside and then back. This is normal embryonic metabolism and also explains how traumatic stress can shift a midline out of the body because the capacity to do so is inherent to the embryo. This is perhaps a much broader definition of the fulcrum and the midline than the reader is familiar with. This is because it is based on the perceptual experience of the practitioner's body first rather than client palpation and secondarily guided by the early stages of development of the embryo.

Thus, the way I currently perceive the healing and therapeutic properties of the embryonic fulcrums and midline is as the *rhythmic balanced interchange* between Primary Respiration and Dynamic Stillness that seeks to expand three dimensionally and reveal its wholeness in a myriad of different perceptions within the various zones. This interchange is a deep therapeutic pulse in the fluid body. This interchange can be expressed differently depending on the zone and the mindfulness and awareness of the practitioner at any given moment in a session. It is not limited to a single rate such as Primary Respiration. In the biodynamic model I teach, however, and given the state of the contemporary client, slower and quiet are more valuable rates and pulses. One teacher once said to just *wait, watch, and wonder*. Perhaps this is the essence of the therapeutic relationship. Practically however, at the end of a session, the client's pulse rate should not be faster than when the session started.

The rhythmic balanced interchange, as Dr. Becker called it, is the biodynamic engine and pulse of life. One or the other qualities of stillness and Primary Respiration is always in the foreground or background of a normal ignition-fulcrum-midline experience. The biodynamic attention process of orienting, synchronizing, attuning, and disengaging is the foundation for establishing this perceptual process. It is the very core of biodynamic healing. It is not an "idle dream," as Dr. Sutherland said. My first three volumes go into quite a bit of detail about this.

Combustion

Another point here in clinical practice is that the practitioner cannot rely on the client's body to have an active, functioning fulcrum-midline inside of it, because the embryonic fulcrums existed outside of the body in their initial development. This is normal and definitions of what constitutes embodiment must be revised. In other words, the organizing fulcrums of the urogenital system, umbilicus, heart, and third ventricle are designed to be displaced or automatically shift between zones A, B, C, and D. It is of vital importance that the practitioner be able to orient and synchronize her attention with the interchange of Primary Respiration and stillness, as it might be located in any or all of the zones. The practitioner takes the pulse of all the zones by shifting attention. Furthermore, I differentiate between combustion, ignition, and initiation, illustrated in Figure 9.1. Ignition exists on a continuum of perceptual experiences as stated. Ignition and its perception are limited without an understanding of how traumatic stress and complex inflammatory conditions cause the body to have uncontained combustion and literally burn up with too much speed or too much inflammation, as discussed in the first four chapters of this book.

Traumatic stress creates a highly volatile metabolism in the fluid body called inflammation. Complex inflammatory conditions are epidemic in the contemporary client. This is why it is important to review the first four chapters to begin to understand how an unhealthful diet promotes inflammation that results in a host of symptoms, disorders, and diseases. As a result of inflammation, the fluid body actually feels dense like tissue without an orientation to a fulcrum or one that is weak, at best. Perceptually, the pulse of the client's fluid body feels fast, erratic, and unorganized. On the other end of the continuum, ignition must be available to and a part of the larger dimension of the deep healing process called *initiation.* Combustion must be contained in order for deep healing to occur.

Initiation

The definition of *initiation,* according to the Third International Webster's Dictionary, is "the rites, ceremonies, ordeals, or instructions with which one is invested with a particular function, especially healing from a disease or illness." Initiation, in the sense that I am using it, thus refers to the nature of a therapeutic session as a healing ceremony or a set of instructions given by Primary Respiration and stillness to the client via the attunement of the practitioner. Proper attunement by the practitioner in the ceremony involves the creation of sacred space that produces a correct realignment with the forces of nature (zone D) for the client. Sacred space is well-bounded space known as a *container* in which the strong forces necessary for transformation can function safely. The strong forces referred to here are fear, depression, and anger. They must be transformed through body awareness and the interchange of Primary Respiration and stillness over time. This is simply a metaphor for zone activity in biodynamic practice, conscious awareness of such zone activity including the practitioner's own body, and how she manages its relationship to ignition or combustion.

Sacred space is further defined as having an organizing middle through which spiritual healing energy comes through to the client. This is the spiritual midline. In biodynamic practice, the spiritual is represented by the natural world and its horizon with the interchange of Primary Respiration and stillness moving back and forth to the practitioner. This is zone D. Remember that zone

D can be all of the earth below the floor and not just nature, the horizon, and the sky out the window. There are moments when the interchange between Primary Respiration and Dynamic Stillness feels like grace, bliss, and joy, no matter which direction they come from. Many clients have commented on the sense of a divine presence entering the room. In this way, the practitioner is a manager of the sacred space as much as a practitioner of manual therapy. This is an important aesthetic in biodynamic practice.

In contemporary biodynamic practice using this metaphor of initiation, the practitioner *is* the organizing center of sacred space. The zones become the container. They are the sacred space. A return to wholeness is the fruition. The entire body-mind perceptual field of the practitioner *is* a spiritual principle, so to speak. This is especially relevant because of the new science of interpersonal neurobiology, which focuses on empathy and compassion. Empathy and compassion are now known to be enhanced by the practitioner's somatic awareness. This necessitates a significant amount of time spent in every session with the practitioner sensing her own body and zone phenomena. I like to suggest to students what I call the 80-20 rule. Start with 80 percent of the time in a session listening to your own body and the zones and devote 20 percent of the time listening to the client with your hands. Gradually this ratio shifts and changes.

The practitioner needs to be able to differentiate or discern between a *stage* of combustion that is capable of being transformed into the *stage* of ignition. Then discernment is made on how ignition is transformed into a *state* of initiation through attention on the interchange function of the fulcrum-midline, the zones, the metabolic fields in the client, and so forth. The client is incubating his own healing as the practitioner manages the space. All management means is the conscious perception of Primary Respiration and stillness through the zones. The practitioner cannot possibly know the specific focus of the client's dilemma at a spiritual level. Some clients live in a sea of unbearable sorrow. She can track the process of healing with Primary Respiration and stillness and take the pulse of the client's fluid body at the beginning, middle, and end of the session to track progress toward a breathing wholeness with Primary Respiration. This is great compassion.

Transitions

As mentioned at the beginning of this chapter, different ignitions are named for specific transitions that occur during life. Thus ignition can also be defined as the power and energy necessary to successfully manage life transitions such as conception, birth, and death. Embryologically, another important transition is the development of the heart and the blood. Consequently, the term *heart ignition* is also found in biodynamic literature and I have written about this in my Volume Three. *Death ignition* is a term mentioned by some practitioners specifically relating to the potency necessary to physically die naturally or the surrender necessary for the dissolving of the self as the body is fading. Death ignition then moves into a phase of spiritual transformation.

From a clinical point of view, whenever a client is going through an important life transition, no matter what age, there is a significant amount of potency available in order to ignite a successful transition to the next phase of life or death. Biodynamic practitioners can borrow from the understanding of developmental psychology in which numerous crises that all people experience are considered normal and necessary transitions from one mode of being to another. This transition energy is frequently squandered, medicated, suppressed, denied, or wasted and thus ignition and its potential for transformation are lost.

A common principle of pre- and perinatal psychology is that the strength and/or severity of a life transition frequently (if not always) is a recapitulation of pre-conception events, or prenatal events such as conception, heart development, and birth. For example, maternal stress alters placental development. Altered placental development frequently leads to obesity, heart disease, and diabetes. This is recapitulation at a metabolic level. Altered placental development also leads to low birth weight and the necessity of a medicalized birth, which interferes with the normal life transition of birth. I watched how the nursing home my mother lived in did everything possible to interfere and deny her dying process. These are just a few examples of normal transitions being thwarted. Thus it is critically important for a client to be held in wholeness with Primary Respiration and stillness so the thwarted and botched transitions in life can be normalized. This is the principle intention of the biodynamic ceremony: you are normal and you are whole and there is only happiness right now.

> The off-center, in-between state is an ideal situation, a situation in which we don't get caught and we can open our hearts and minds beyond limit. To stay with that shakiness—to stay with a broken heart, for example, or with a rumbling stomach, with a feeling of hopelessness or wanting to get revenge—is to stay on the path of true awakening. Sticking with that uncertainty, getting the knack of relaxing in the midst of chaos, learning not to panic—this is the spiritual path.
>
> (Chodron, 2011, p. 16)

Physical illness and disease can be looked at as having a spiritual cause in the sense that disease is a disconnection from the living wholeness of the zones acting as one thing. This is another reason why the change process inherent in life transitions is frequently characterized as terrifying and fearful. This is precisely the energy that needs to be surrendered to and transformed into a new way or mode of being for both the practitioner and the client. It is because of this deep sense of terror and fear that traditional cultures created healing ceremonies and initiatory processes to manage this level of ignition and avoid too much combustion and premature death. Sometimes it takes a community to help one person get realigned and in proper relationship with the forces of nature and a spiritual purpose. Clinically, the practitioner needs to focus on working from her zone B to the client's zone B after stabilizing one's perception in zones A, C, and D. Biodynamic practice holds the client in his totality including the pre-conception dynamic that is a major influence on health and well-being. I highly recommend that the practitioner have a spiritual practice and make a commitment to self-care. Compassion always begins with one's own self.

Summary

The clinical intention in general is for the practitioner to be able to recognize ignition by paying attention to her own buoyant three dimensionality, the interchange between Primary Respiration and stillness, the events that occur during the two phases of Primary Respiration, and discerning the value and meaning of various zone phenomena and whether they relate to the healing process. This includes working zone B to zone B when it is available by focusing on the stillness in zone B. This is biodynamic multitasking. At first the practitioner learns each of these as a separate practice and gradually they become a seamless continuum with the help of Primary Respiration. Then they become one unified pulse in the fluid body manifesting harmony. Primary Respiration is what directs the attention of the practitioner.

It is simply too much to pay attention to everything mentioned here or any book written on the subject of ignition and fulcrum-midline, including my other volumes. What gradually emerges is that the practitioner self-regulates at her own pace using the important biodynamic principle of waiting patiently for Primary Respiration and stillness to show the way. Then comes watching them manifest their priorities, and then feeling the wonder of the biodynamic process. While waiting, gradually the interchange between Primary Respiration and stillness may be recognized as the balance of life and death constantly occurring right now in the body. This balance is known not by being able to always perceive a fifty-second tidal rhythm and its direction, but rather by the emergence of *life-affirming qualities*. The life-affirming qualities of love, happiness, joy, kindness, bliss, equanimity, patience, generosity, and more become woven into the fabric of everyday life and clinical practice. This to me is the true wonder of biodynamic practice. It is grace unfolding.

As I have already said, ignition refers to events and processes that cause a continual transition to wholeness as a living, buoyant, bodily experience. It is through ignition that people create meaning for their life. Ignition is thus a cause for joy and lightheartedness and is a necessity for a differentiated wholeness that keeps on integrating life and bodily experience. Primary Respiration cannot be underestimated in its value and intention.

Biodynamic sessions do not end with Primary Respiration or having a buoyant fluid body. I would like to suggest that there is no ending nor beginning, just an ongoing affirmation of life with qualities that were always already present and just become uncovered through the process of slowing, stilling, and attending to the natural world of the mind and body three dimensionally. In the end we become lighthearted and engage life wholeheartedly. Our heart shows signs of a stronger pulse that extends beyond the body in all directions.

CHAPTER 10

Holographic Touch™: Engaging the Continuum of Consciousness

by Carol A. Agneessens, MS

Two questions have captured my passion and curiosity over the thirty-five-plus years I have practiced in the healing arts. The first question: *What is a body?* And the second: If our bodies are the physical expression of something bigger than a personal self, *how do I touch all that a body is?*

This chapter is based on the sensory experience that we are "whole" from the very beginning of life. It is this wholeness that health care practitioners are able to contact and that is key in sustaining a transformational process. This implicit oneness is charged with the potency of consciousness imbuing all living things.

The idea of whole, a unit, the undivided, is foreign to our culture and is slowly vanishing like an aboriginal form that is viewed as "primitive" by the intellect. Each one of us faces the reality in ourselves and must meet that responsibility first, and then the perception will follow (Jealous, 1997).

In my desire to know and touch the spectrum of consciousness expressed through the varying densities within and around our physical bodies, I slowly came to the realization that the quality of my touch echoes my state of mind. By cultivating an ability to shift my awareness, through attention to perceptual cues and body sensation, I am able to more clearly listen and sense the unseen dimensions of an individual's system. Through the medium of my hands, as an extension of my heart and body knowing, I've discovered that quietly sitting and waiting at the edges of someone's body space cultivates a perceptual synaesthesia, allowing me to feel-touch-see and gain a clearer sense of the person's systemic voice. In a state of quiet receptivity, I am learning to listen.

Holographic Touch[1] asks the health care practitioner to attend to his or her own perceptions, somatic feedback, and state of mind, instead of directing focus entirely toward the other. As you will see and feel, when attention is given to our own perceptions and sensorium, a portal opens to an exquisite gestalt:

state of consciousness → quality of touch → multidimensional → somatic[2] awakening

The following inquiries are designed to initiate an exploration regarding your familiar patterns of engaging through touch. Take a moment to consider the following questions.

How Do You Begin a Session?

As you ask yourself the following questions, notice the body sensations generated by your response.

- Do you begin your session with focus and intention on the expressed problem?

- Do you begin your session with an intention, goal, or idea about the desired outcome?

- Do you engage as a participant in a process of transformation or as the "doer," holding the responsibility of fixing the problem?

- Is the majority of your attention directed into your client or do you maintain a sense of yourself in the session?

The alchemy of touch and presence is a potent elixir. Holographic Touch cultivates receptivity to the many dimensions of consciousness. By questioning firmly held beliefs about healing, and the nature of our physical reality, we can expand the boundaries of our own perceiving field. It is possible to engage with this underlying plenum of consciousness, interconnectivity, and the original blueprint of the body. It is our own *perceptual armoring* that blinds us to the multidimensional rhythms of life that are already there yet buried under the flurry of thoughts and activity.

---

1. Holographic: The condition upon which the information for creating a whole system is stored in each of its parts. Through the application of a coherent light source, a three-dimensional image is recreated from the memory of wholeness held in each of the parts. (From lycaeum.org)

2. In this context I am using the word *somatic* to refer to the continuum of manifest consciousness expressing through the physical.

There is no place in this new kind of physics both for the field and matter, for the field is the only reality.

(Albert Einstein)

Within the imagined solidity of the body exists vast spaciousness. Our bodies are a temporary expression of the mystery that we call life.

When scientists study complex systems, the notion of parts begins to break down so that *quantification* of such systems becomes impossible.... By contrast, in *qualitative* measurement, plots show the shape of the system's movements as a whole.

(Briggs and Peat, 1989, pp. 83–85)

Sitting within the quiet flow of Primary Respiration, our hands engage with the physical expression of consciousness—the body—and witness the shape-changing effects of this rhythm throughout. A three-dimensional spaciousness expands beyond the boundary of skin. The intelligence within consciousness is greater than the matter of our flesh.

What we observe as material bodies and forces are nothing but shapes and variations in the structure of space.

(Erwin Schrodinger)

A dynamic pulse of stillness vivifies the center of a nonmaterial and translucent midline. Within a spacious interior, a numinous thread arises, a "line" of vibrating potential, weaving together cosmos and earth, organizing, informing, yet not penetrating the body's density.

Man is something organized around a line.

(Ida P. Rolf)

The Dynamic of Touch and Consciousness: Efferent and Afferent Perceptual Styles

In the ever quickening pace of a world squeezed by schedules and deadlines of time, the seduction of "doing" chains many to watching the clock. Self-worth is often keyed to what we effect or accomplish in an hour or compress into a day. These patterns are reflected in nervous system activity and create a perceptual bias and tonal resonance.

To *effect* something is to change the state as a direct result of action by doing. *Efferent* perception radiates awareness like a force field in order to sense the environment. This is a field of vigilance (Ridley, 2006, p. 22). It is a model for directing intention into a system in order to correctly palpate, find the cause, and resolve it.

> Efference is derived from thinking, objectifying, separating, planning, and wanting to know what is going on in your client's body. Any perception, touch, technique, intention, or preconceived idea of motion that you apply to your client is efferent.
>
> (Ridley, 2006, pp. 186–187)

Afferent perception describes attention inwardly directed. This is a state of receptivity to being in-formed. It is a state of yielding into the unknown moment. In this place of "not-doing," the systemic intelligence of another informs the practitioner. Afference requires waiting. I have found that an individual's system "speaks" most clearly to me if I wait at the edges of the person's skin boundary attending to my own orientations, sensations, and perceptions. I wait and wait, and wait a little more as the person's system becomes acquainted with the tonal resonance of my presence and, like a deer in the forest, begins to understand that the one who is waiting is not predator and he or she is not prey.

> Touch has an effect on different centers of the brain, but especially the insular cortex. This part of the OFC (orbital frontal cortex) is generally regarded as having self-regulatory control of the entire corticolimbic system and autonomic nervous system. This means that the client who is receiving physical contact is unconsciously reading the context of the touch as much as the sensation of the touch.
>
> (Shea, 2008, p. 202)

The ability to differentiate whether we are touching and perceiving with an efferent or an afferent perceptual resonance is essential for cultivating receptivity in our hands and our touch. The fight-flight-freeze response inflamed by an efferent tone is quieted. As I continue to gain clarity about the subtle yet profound shifts in body sensation and state of mind between these two perceptual styles, the following inquiry arose.

Inquiry: Identifying Your Perceptual Style

As you sit in a comfortably aligned position, notice where your attention is settling. Notice if your attention moves easily out into the space around you or rests within yourself and your own body skin, or do you perceive a little of both—being out and being in at the same time?

1. Notice the quality of your body sensations as you intentionally direct your attention into the room around you, directing it at a picture or plant or thing in the room.

   Notice the felt sense of extending your attention specifically toward another person, whether he or she is in the room with you or in another place.

   Notice any shifting sensation in your cranium, your eyes, and your breath as you direct your attention, as if it is a force field toward another. This is efferent perception.

2. Settle into a sense of body orientation—a sense of your feet on the floor, and the space around you. Perhaps you experience a sense of the weight of your body being supported by the chair as well as a soft visual sense of the room you are in. Imagine a center of stillness deep within the midline of your body. Allow your intention to rest in that center of stillness.

   Allow the sounds in the room to come to you. If you hear a bird singing, allow the sound outside the window to come to you.

   If you can imagine being with a close friend, notice how it feels to settle into the security of your friendship, waiting for the friend to share the insights of his or her life. This exchange has the quality of afference.

Describe the difference you experience between these two perceptual styles.

As a dedicated practitioner of structural integration for many years, my work was informed by anatomical drawings, dissection labs, reading, and workshops guided by efferent perception. This is the Newtonian body and biomechanical anatomy.[3] It was important to have this lens in order to correctly palpate, find the cause of the stated structural problem, and resolve it. It was imperative to know and understand the function, anatomy, and integral structure of the body. With this anatomical background, many pain symptoms and client concerns were relieved.

Anatomy, especially when studied through the remains of a dry cadaver, reveals the biomechanical underpinnings of the Newtonian body. Classically, it was thought that this body was a machine. If it is broken, it can be fixed, either by replacing a part (as in modern-day surgery) or putting a part in a better place for more efficient movement. A Newtonian view employs a fix-it model of the world. And in this state of mind, it works.

---

3. Although the descriptions I offer relating to the spectrum of consciousness and physical densities are different, I acknowledge Emilie Conrad for inspiring these classifications.

However, when I touch, guided by Netter's *Illustrated Anatomy* as both map and template, my hands become more tool-like and I work from a mechanical linearity. Often, in an attempt to address the identified problem (the particulate structure embedded in connective tissue), or in my zeal to find IT and fix IT, the "lesion" being investigated blocks the movement of an interconnecting wave. The joy of years in the field of structural integration occurred when anatomical knowledge receded and I was guided by a systemic intelligence lighting the way through the myofascial planes.

> Like the mass points of Newton, humans appear to be self-contained, mutually independent chunks of organized matter only externally related to each other and to their environment.
>
> (Ervin Lazlo)

Inquiry: Touch and the Biomechanical Mind

The exploration described here is not about your knowledge of anatomy but about attention to shifts in your state of mind, perceptions, and quality of touch when you are focused on palpating a specific anatomical part. What is your experience as you search for and palpate a particular anatomical structure, whether it is gross anatomy or delicate nerve fibers? Notice the qualitative shifts as you assume the intentional mind behind palpatory specificity.

1. Sit beside a partner; place your hand on your partner's thigh.
2. Focus your intention on contacting the middle of the rectus femoris muscle. Remember the anatomical picture of the muscle beneath your hand. Let your hands palpate the musculature. When your attention focuses on a particular "event" (in this instance we call the event the rectus femoris), what do you notice happens to the felt-sense of your hand?
3. How does your partner experience your touch?

Try this a few more times with different anatomical landmarks, perhaps bone or organ or ligament. Attend to the quality of your touch.

When my intention is to palpate or manipulate specific tissues, with the efferent tone of fixing, I lose a quality of curiosity, a gentle inquiring into the unknown territory of another and the subtle exchange that occurs when I take the time, not only to touch, but to be touched by another's somatic intelligence. Is it possible to set aside the belief that depth is a matter of muscle or directing intention into another's body? Whether you are diving into tissues with a strong hand or an energetic one, notice the quality of your touch, your thoughts, and the felt sense of your own system as you work from a Newtonian understanding of the body.

> I do not see anatomy when I treat. I do not visualize, yet I see a physiological living process in motion. Visualization of static anatomy inhibits function in both the operator and the patient. Let the process reveal itself to all your senses, you will "see" clearly.
>
> (Jim Jealous)

Sensing Fluidity: The Embryonic Body and Primordial Anatomy

> A successful response from the cerebrospinal fluid … is an intensified interchange between all the fluids of the body…. It is definitely evident that the reaction is systemic and includes the whole body even within the bones.
>
> (Anne Wales, DO)

There is an ocean within. A saline viscosity permeates every nook and cranny of our body—floating cells, vessels, organs, and bones. Contained by the boundary of skin, fluids generate pathways of information flow, connectivity, and conductivity. The sacred waters within our body space carry life's beginnings emerging from the primordial well of time.

The Scientific Basis for a Fluid Body

As my thinking shifts from a fix-it state of mind to one of fluid integration, a homogenous quality can be sensed throughout the physical body. Bones, blood, lymph, nerve, musculature, etc. share one coherent movement. Fluidity engenders the sensation of wholeness.

William Sutherland, DO, the founder of cranial osteopathy, spoke of a fluid body that held the lesions of a system and obstructed movement toward an individual's well-being. The relationship between the physical and the fluid body is really the foundation of the biodynamics and biokinetics of embryology (Jealous, 2000).

The embryo, as an archetype of perfect form, serves as a blueprint for our body's ability to heal itself. The formative and regenerative *fluid forces* that organize embryological development are present throughout our life span, ready for our cooperation in harnessing their therapeutic potency. In other words, the forces of embryogenesis become the forces of healing after birth (McPartland and Skinner, 2005, pp. 22–32).

During childhood, water comprises a significant proportion of our bodies (75–80 percent). As adults our total body water decreases to about 60 percent. Bones are 20 percent fluid (Rosen, 2008). Unpublished research at the Max Planck Institute, however, suggests that the percentage of fluid in the body may be as high as 92 percent.

Our bodies are mostly fluid. Although as adults it is said that we lose this as we age, remember that once upon a time we were a fluid and pulsating mass of undifferentiated potential in the saline sea of a maternal womb. Initially, 98 percent of the embryo is fluid. It is this fluid movement that lays down the shape for muscles, bones, and other anatomical structures. Water knows no boundary and in an enclosed system spiraling patterns imprint all function and structure.

Living tissues contain thousands of different kinds of molecules, each of which is surrounded by water. Most people do not recognize that the body is a water system that both regulates and conducts information and can be imprinted with stress. Molecules do not have to touch each other to interact.

> The electromagnetic field along with water forms the matrix of life. Water can form structures that transmit energy.
>
> (Oschman, 2000, p. 60)

The fluid body, as named by James Jealous, DO, shapes and reshapes texture and form. This body resonates with life-perpetuating potency and is a unique biological entity. To engage the fluid body of another, I must be willing to engage this dimension permeating and surrounding my own physical body. Spiraling and interconnecting fluidity moves through me, softening and melting the density of structural compressions held by the ground substance of flesh. Porous and permeable, my sensorium expands as I engage a different kind of knowing and remembering.

I dwell in primordial waters. Sitting within this fluidic egg, my mind shifts from linear patterns of thinking to an instinctual knowing. Inspiration infuses and ignites cortical firings and glial connections, from cause-effect to acausal understanding, from isolation to connection with something more than that which I know myself to be.

In this world, the edges soften and something "other" breathes me. Fluid conducts and carries information. These oceanic inner waters of life sustain a deepening harmony crucial to health and connectivity.

According to the Bushman, an individual's separation from that part of one's self that is connected to "everything else" leads to fear and a sense of aloneness, and this facilitates the disease process. Because treatment using the BOCF (biodynamic osteopathy in the cranial field) connects the patient to nature, the patient receives an immediate experience of "not-aloneness" or "belonging" in a deep way (McPartland and Skinner, 2005).

If I wish to sense and know the fluid body I must cultivate an afferent way of knowing and touching. As a practitioner, I have to reduce the cultural bias driving efferent activity. I have to question the intention I direct through an individual's system and yield to the sensory understanding of a receptive perceptual state of mind.

Inquiry: Engaging the Fluid Body

This exploration is in three parts. Initially it is important to get feedback on the familiar way you initially contact another when you begin a session.

1. Sit side by side a partner. Place your "working" hand on your partner's thigh.

   How do you experience the touch of your own hand? How does your partner experience your touch? Give and receive feedback.

2. Sense your buoyant hand. In your own hand, sense its inner ocean. Allow your awareness to rest within the bones of your hand; settle into the blood-filled lattices of your bone marrow. Take time to sensually absorb the transformation of your hand as you remember its inherent fluidity.

3. Now, place your fluid hand on your partner's thigh. Explore the felt sense of your hand as a buoyant medium, floating on the sea of interstitial fluids and tissues comprising your partner's thigh.

   Do you and/or your partner experience a different quality in your contact when you initiate with a fluid hand rather than your familiar hand?

   With a buoyant hand, do you or your partner experience a contact that engages the whole?

As practitioner, do you notice any shift in your perception or state of mind as you sense more of your own fluidic nature? Perhaps there is a slowing down, a sense of relaxation, or some other shift in perception as you sense the fluidity of your hand.

Notice if instead of feeling only muscle you may feel the homogeneity of your partner's (or client's) body. For example, the bones, tissues, and fluids feel interconnected, as if they are one thing.

Allow a sense of the back of your hand as much as the palm surface that is in contact with your partner.

Try this a few more times with different anatomical landmarks, perhaps bone or organ or ligament. Attend to your quality of touch and the shift in state of body-mind.

The fluid body remains hidden from my perception when I engage "it" from a biomechanical state of mind, or as a technique to be applied when all else fails. It is a whole-body experience of becoming one, of embracing both our autonomy and connectedness to everything at one and the same time. It is a practice of knowing this duality yet releasing it in order to be taken to a ground of wholeness in which the ego-driven self is no longer the one who knows or is the doer.

> There is no drop of water in the ocean, not even in the deepest parts of the abyss, that does not know and respond to the mysterious forces that create the tide.
>
> (Rachel Carson)

The Quantum Body: Engaging the Holographic Matrix

As practitioners in the healing arts, we have the rare opportunity to remember our interconnectedness to a world beyond our brain and body. The potential for perceiving multidimensionality arises in each therapeutic session. The sensorial understanding, that our bodies are the portal through which we engage dimensions beyond the scientifically proven or physically manifest, is an ever-present reality. In Western culture, these dimensions are often ridiculed, dismissed, and denied. Our bodies are a condensation of consciousness—a range of knowledge exists through and beyond the physical realm.

Consciousness extends in all directions throughout all matter of space and time. In order to experience these multidimensional facets, I have worked through my own perceptual barriers cultivating the somatic qualities of permeability and fluidity. In a very real sense, accessing this domain requires a reexamination of my beliefs about what the body is and ways of living. By exploring beyond the culturally myopic view of how life functions, a realization and understanding emerges igniting a unified field of knowing. We can remember our fundamental wholeness, a beginning that speaks to an inseparable connection to everyone and everything.

How is it that we can learn to touch in a way that supports the remembering of origins and the underlying matrix that is cosmic consciousness? Our hands can become a vibrating continuum between the most solidified forms of consciousness (like bone) to the more subtle forms of consciousness—the original matrix, the informational field, and the rich emptiness that holds all. In order to immerse myself in this phenomenal field, I was jolted by the realization that this continuum is always there. It was my own perceptual armoring that restricted this sensual knowing.

Although I was introduced to the geodesic dome of Buckminster Fuller's genius years ago, it was only recently and while walking the beach during winter's low tide that an image of an iridescent blue tensegrity shape appeared before me. This image flashed as if it were neon. I hurried home to research the cellular existence of the structure. Tensegrity proffered an explanation for the unusual visual and kinesthetic feedback arising through my hands during biodynamic craniosacral sessions. And it was the exceedingly fine interlinked filaments forming the cellular geodesic structures that I sensed and envisioned in my hands.

Triangular, octahedral, and tetrahedral forms are self-organizing patterns in all biological structures. They represent the best organization of least energy (energy-efficient) and mass (size) through structures of continuous tension and local compression, that is, through tensegrity (Volokh, Vilnay, and Belsky, 2002).

Throughout his numerous writings, Ervin Laszlo speaks of a cosmic memory field. He defines this as a real, lived experience that conveys a thought, an image, or an intuition that was not transmitted by our senses either at the time it happened or at any time before. This lived experience occurs in the extra- or nonsensory mode (Laszlo, 2009). Perhaps I had entered Laszlo's field of cosmic envisioning during my twilight walk.

Inquiry: Your Multidimensional Hand and Holographic Touch

This inquiry is first done solo and then with a partner who is lying on a table.

1. A solo exploration: Notice the shape and felt sense of your hand. Let it rest on your thigh.

    Sense the texture of your clothing on which your hand rests. Let your attention rest in the surface of your palm (as if your palm could count the threads of your clothing).

    Now sense the space in the middle of your hand. That is the space of bone, blood, tissues, and fluids. Allow a sense of depth and dimension in your hand.

    As you settle and sense the field around you, notice and allow the back of your hand gently expanding away from your palm, which remains in contact with the clothing of your thigh.

Notice the spacious dimensionality within your hand. You might feel the entire inside space of your hand as fluid and breathing.

Do not "will" this experience. Just notice the response in your hand as you recognize the dimensions of your inside space.

2. Now, with your partner: Settle yourself in a place of quiet stillness. Comfortably sit so that you are facing the side of your partner (at waist level).

Place your lower hand underneath your partner's thigh or knee (whichever is more comfortable for your arm extension) and your upper hand beneath his or her shoulder. This is a position called the Pietà (Shea, 2005).

Settle into an awareness of the contact between the palm surface of your hand and your partner. Allow this perception to deepen as you sense the whole of his or her system.

Notice the space between your palm and the back of your hand. You may begin to sense expansion through the tissues in the middle of your hand. It may feel as if the back of your hand is expanding away from the surface of your palm.

Wait. (An important caveat in all explorations: *Do not* drive the exploration through will or a concept of what you imagine is supposed to happen. Wait; let your system find the sensory qualities of expansion, space, and breath.)

As you wait in this state of deepening stillness, cultivate a sense of the field around you, containing and holding you. You do not have to go out to find it. Instead, become aware of the ever-present and potent field surrounding and permeating you. Perceive even the most subtle shifts within your hand and perceiving self. You might begin to notice the back of your hand slowly extending into the field—perhaps meeting the edges of the room or even beyond the room.

As you experience your hands becoming more permeable, continue to notice the deepening stillness and connection that is occurring between you, your partner, and the field. You may experience a moment where the membranes of separation dissolve. You might also notice that your partner's body is becoming more porous and following the movement of spacious connection into the field.

While exploring Holographic Touch, I realized that my touch needed to be more than a feather's weight. As I engage an individual's system—with gentle yet firm presence—my hands began to transform in the distinct way I have described. They became more porous and dimensional, and my client's system mirrored this state. Whether I was connecting with organ, tissue, or bone, I experienced the synesthesia of seeing-feeling the individual's system expanding into the vast field surrounding both of us. The membranes separating his or her system, my system, my hands, his or her issues, became a unified experience of expansion, and shifting form. From these experiences, the role of the tensegrity function was clarified. I imagine it to be the archetypal functional-structure connecting the intercellular space of my body's trillion-plus cells to the holographic matrix and blueprint of origin. Tensegrity lifts the compressive forces of cultural imprinting, trauma and injury.

From the palpable and experiential to the scientifically researched, I found that cellular tensegrity provides both a sensorial bridge and biological understanding for the continuum I was experiencing. The body as a whole and the matrix we are embedded within form a geodesic continuum. In a way it is the gossamer glue of our cosmic connectedness.

A tensegrity structure forms a stable yet dynamic system that interacts efficiently and resiliently with forces acting upon it. Tensegrity provides a conceptual link between the structural systems and the energy-informational systems (Oschman, 2000).

> Cells and intracellular elements are capable of vibrating in a dynamic manner with complex harmonics, the frequency of which can now be measured and analyzed.... It is important to understand the mechanism by which this vibrational information is transferred directly throughout the cell. From these observations we propose that vibrational information is transferred through a tissue tensegrity-matrix.... A tensegrity tissue matrix system allows for specific transfer of information through the cell by direct transmission of vibrational chemomechanical energy through harmonic wave motion.
>
> (Coffey and Pienta, 1991)

Summary

Sitting in the stillness of the mystery we call life, I recognize the subtle yet palpable dimensions just beyond the seductive veil of the material world.

By following my passion to expand the spectrum of my touch, I found my way to Holographic Touch and its ignition of a numinous body. By questioning the belief that diving into physiological depths is the avenue for repair, a novel understanding arose. Waiting at the edges, orienting to my own sensorium, and cultivating spaciousness within my own hand-body space reveal another way of healing that fosters dimensionality within the other. A holographic touch yields the recognition of the ONE that is embracing us all. By engaging the infinitely fine tissues, functions, and structures of the body, the often compressive imprints of our origins, birth, injury, and society can be lifted.

Remembering that our bodies are one with and embedded in a cosmic plenum touches a kinesthetic knowing; the marrow of our bones flows with the marrow of the holographic matrix. Lymph, blood, and fluids stream through our bodies, as cosmic intelligence streams through all existence. The breath of Primary Respiration breathes us all.

We talk about the mind-body field as if they were separate but, in fact, it is our attention that is split.

Imagining there is a difference between my inside self and outside, I return again and again to the felt realization of seamlessness. I touch another and I am touched. I perceive consciousness in life and I am perceived by consciousness itself.

> My hand is able to touch things only because my hand is a touchable thing…. Similarly, the eyes with which I see things are themselves visible…. to touch the coarse skin of a tree is thus at the same time to experience one's own tactility, to feel oneself touched by the tree. And to see the world is also, at the same time, to experience oneself as visible, to feel oneself seen.
>
> (Abram, 1996, p. 68)

Reprinted with permission from Carol A. Agneessens.

CHAPTER 11

Ten Steps to Client Participation in Biodynamic Practice

Getting the Client Involved

This chapter explores the theory and practice of teaching the client how to participate in the biodynamic therapeutic process. It is a critical component in biodynamic practice. My friend Sarajo Berman calls the therapeutic relationship "joint practice." It is known from the field of interpersonal neurobiology that the therapeutic relationship is a two-person biology. The brains and hearts of two people in relationship are mirroring and matching each other, especially regarding feelings and emotions. This requires that the practitioner become much more aware of his or her own body. By spending a majority of time gently concentrating on the practitioner's own wholeness and three dimensionality at a sensory level, a resonance for the client's nervous and vascular systems is generated to do the same. This reorients both nervous systems to a slow tempo and periodic stillness that is essential for growth, development, empathy, compassion, and happiness.

On the one hand, the therapeutic relationship in biodynamic practice is centered on the perceptual processes of the practitioner. On the other hand, it becomes vitally important to get clients involved in developing their own biodynamic practice before, during, and after a session. This is the new balance in the therapeutic relationship. The client needs to be taught how to participate in his or her own healing process. The therapeutic relationship from this point of view is a form of communion as well as communication. It depends more upon clients giving feedback to the practitioner about how the session unfolds in their life than it does upon practitioners telling clients what is going on in their body.

While some practitioners may have this habit and even be accurate at times, it may have an element of projection from the practitioner onto the client, and possibly wishful thinking. I try to stay as neutral as possible and keep my comments very general. I can report to a client what type of rhythms I might be experiencing in his or her body without it being interpretive or judgmental. And, yes, I will occasionally tell the client that I have felt "progress." I am very careful when I do so.

To balance biodynamic craniosacral therapy with a client-centered approach, the client needs to be able to sense his or her own body and especially the slow tidal movements causing the three-dimensional shape of the body to constantly change. This may result in stress reduction and what I like to call happiness induction.

The biggest challenge with the contemporary client is the lack of embodiment from an overactive autonomic nervous system (ANS). This results in a body that carries too much speed and fear. In order to build safety into the relationship, the client must be empowered to participate. Because the ANS has strong resistance to slowing down, the client needs to feel and know the value of slowing and stilling. The resistance may at times feel uncomfortable, and this needs to be expressed by the client. The client will have his or her own metaphor to describe the experience and the practitioner must listen for it. It is simply based on the known value of consciously slowing and stilling, unplugging from the internet (physically or metaphorically), and supporting the client to move through any discomfort by using any of the skills in the ten-step process described below. The important somatic education and a principal component of biodynamic practice as I teach it.

The Steps

Slowing and stilling requires balancing two kinds of attention: focused attention (left hemisphere of the brain) and unfocused attention (right hemisphere of the brain). Within those two kinds of attention, there are skills involving a slow tempo, breathing, and three-dimensional awareness that can facilitate a much deeper level of healing when the client participates. I have put together a ten-step set of guidelines for the practitioner to teach or coach clients in order to solicit their involvement before, during, and after sessions. The ten steps are as follows:

1. Create the shared intention of a joint practice with the client.

2. Teach the client the *gift* of a body scan in a supine position on the table.

3. Introduce the vehicle of breath as a way to deepen the experience of the body scan.

4. Teach the client how to synchronize the breath with the body and Primary Respiration.

5. Invite reflective awareness.

6. Introduce horizon therapy as another gift, which clients can take from the therapeutic work together.

7. Deepen into horizon therapy by exploring body alignment of the head and neck.

8. Fine-tune the skills of horizon therapy through the client's quality of attention from focused to unfocused.

9. Help the client find his or her heart.

10. Complete the gift of horizon therapy though the therapeutic skill of support. Invite the client to create a time and space in his or her life to practice horizon therapy.

The guiding principle in all these steps is that the practitioner is also performing them on herself or himself, along with the client. It is a restating of a couple of wise old maxims: *Physician heal thyself* and *Do unto others that which you first do unto yourself.*

Let's look at these ten steps in more detail, as I offer some simple how-to suggestions for implementing them.

Step 1: I always start with a new client by giving the complete set of client coaching guidelines verbally. I let clients know that they are expected to dialogue with me about their sensory or bodily experience before a session, as in the case of reporting about their previous session. Sometimes we talk about their experience during a session, especially if they are experiencing some discomfort. I tell my clients that they must let me know if they become uncomfortable or feel any pain or simply want to change position on the table. Sometimes we dialogue at the end of the session, if appropriate, given that most clients are not cognitive immediately after receiving a session.

By informing my clients about these opportunities for dialogue, I create an intention with them for joint practice and naturally evoke the power of empathy and compassion in a two-person biology. The basic work is to feel felt by the other person in order to reduce fear, and this requires a dialogue about sensation and feelings. During any phase of the session, the practitioner is also practicing active listening and reflecting, smiling, and making eye contact. This establishes safety in the therapeutic relationship by helping the client to feel felt by the practitioner.

Step 2: Once the client lies supine on the table at the beginning of a session, I take the first three minutes to practice a body scan with the client without any physical contact. I use a calm, well modulated voice, asking the client to focus his or her attention starting at the feet, and gradually I name the parts of the body all the way up to the top of the client's head. This must be done at a slow tempo—not as one big run-on sentence directing the client. I will participate in this body scan and pause between sentences to practice it on myself. The body scan gives a signal to the nervous system that the body is whole and three-dimensional. It bears repeating in every session.

There are many variations on this theme regarding a body scan. For example, I usually start by asking the client to attend to the surface of the skin as I work my way up the body in the naming of its parts. Or I may, in a follow-up session, ask the client to sense the bones or muscles, starting at the feet. My advice to practitioners is to be creative with the body scan, because the body scan is the foundation of joint practice and is usually done at the beginning of every session. This also becomes a simple homework assignment for clients, that they perform one or two body scans each day when feeling stress or as a way of waking up in the morning and going to bed at night. It builds the felt sense of wholeness and self-regulates stressful experiences.

Step 3: Gradually over several sessions, I invite clients to do a guided relaxation with a focus on their breathing—again, without physical contact between us. This is like a graduate version of the body scan. I ask clients to take a slow, deep, full inhalation and as they exhale to allow their feet and legs to relax and settle more fully on the table. As in step 2, I simply guide clients up to the top of their head verbally. I take big pauses so that clients can breathe for several cycles without instruction. I can also participate by tuning in to my own breathing, between client directives. I generally don't ask clients to do any more than five directed relaxation breaths in this early phase of a session, because the respiratory diaphragm has a very intimate connection with the ANS and it is important to not overstimulate the client's ANS. The key here is gentleness and relaxation.

Step 4: During the session itself, I may periodically ask clients to take a deep breath while I am in contact. Asking clients to breathe is a very important dynamic in the entire lineage of cranial work as it was handed down from Dr. Sutherland. Traditionally, clients would be asked to breathe into the point of contact where the practitioner's hands were located on the client's body, to bring awareness and release to specific tensions in the soft tissue. That is also a valid way to work in biodynamic practice because it will lead to a stable ANS. The biodynamic consideration, however, is to help clients ignite the deeper potencies of order and organization as a function of Primary Respiration. This deeply assists the ignition process in the midline of the client. These potencies of Primary Respiration then permeate the entire body three dimensionally.

I time my request for clients to take a deep breath so that it is synchronized with my perception of the client's Primary Respiration starting its expansion phase. This can be done from any hand position.

As a note of caution, I rarely ask clients to take more than three slow, full-bodied breaths during a session, for the same reason mentioned in step 3. It is very easy for respiration to move from being an ally in the healing process to becoming a defensive strategy. Consequently, the practitioner must be able to sense if the fluid body locks up as a result of asking the client to breathe. I will ask clients to take a deep breath slowly and then track the response in their fluid body for several cycles of their breathing before possibly soliciting another breath. One breath may be all that is necessary to support ignition.

I do not solicit client breathing in every session. I usually wait until we have done at least three sessions. Then I will let the client know before the session begins that I may ask him or her to take a few directed breaths during the session. It is also important to ask the client to breathe several seconds before Primary Respiration is about to change phases and expand. In this way the client inhalation will be more synchronized with the start of the expansion phase of the cycle. This adds fuel to the spark at that point of the ignition process where it is most needed.

Step 5: At the end of a session, I tell the client that I am finished and to please rest for several minutes while I leave and wash my hands. When I return, I sit next to the table and gently ask "How are you?" I may remind clients of the body scan we did at the beginning of the session and ask them to repeat the scan briefly if they report confusion or seem disoriented. Many clients are noncognitive at the end of a session or simply in a state of deep relaxation. If a client gets up too fast, he or she may feel dizzy; physical support may help the client in transitioning slowly. The practitioner needs to assess clients' ability to integrate their experience and be able to drive home. Avoid too many premature questions with clients about what they are feeling at the end of a session. Let clients lead in how they offer sensory information about the session. Of course, some clients are wired to be very talkative almost immediately after a session; in that case I might ask the client to pause and do a silent body scan if he or she seems *too* cognitive. Sometimes, I move into step 6 and wait until that is finished before asking clients about their sensory experience resulting from the session. There really is no set formula except to find ways to support clients in becoming biodynamically involved in their own body.

Step 6: This step begins what is called horizon therapy, which involves a different but related sequence of client coaching guidelines. I prefer to do horizon therapy after the session is over, either in the treatment room or out in the front of my office where the windows are bigger. I inform clients at the beginning of the session that we will take several minutes at the end to do an attention-moving process for brain integration. I do tell them that it is called horizon therapy and it will deepen the work we are doing on the table. I sit in a chair next to the client, who is also seated in a chair.

In this first part of horizon therapy, I place my hands around the front and back of the client's diaphragm. I do a brief body scan, getting the client connected to his or her feet, pelvis, trunk, neck, and head. Then I take a few moments just to sense the client breathing. Next I verbally invite the client's attention to his or her own breathing by saying "Just notice how your breath comes in and out of your nose and mouth. (pause) Now notice how your lungs rise and fall with your rib cage. (pause) Now notice the diaphragm all the way around where my hands are." This may be all that is necessary as breathing is a doorway into Primary Respiration and its various potencies. I ask the client to settle into the breathing between my hands. I like to track five or six breaths and then decide where, when, or how to proceed to the next deepening or to go to the next step with Primary Respiration. If I stay in the tempo of Primary Respiration, then the next phase is simple. The insight will automatically arise in me.

In follow-up sessions I hold the intention to help clients breathe into their abdomen and, specifically, between the umbilicus and the pubic bone. This can dramatically reduce sympathetic fight-flight responses and calm the heart and brain. If a client is not breathing down into the abdomen, I simply place one hand over the umbilicus and my other hand on the client's lower back. With my hands in this position, I invite the client to allow the breath to drop into the abdomen without forcing or pushing. I might suggest to the client to breathe down the front of the spine into my hands. Again, I do not want to be intrusive, so I only practice with five or six cycles of a client's breath. I let the client know that breathing in this location of the body can reduce stress responses in the body by lowering the heart rate.

Step 7: The next phase of horizon therapy is cueing clients for proper placement of the head on the neck. This is for becoming aware of the head-righting reflex, which involves a system of nerves, soft tissue, and proprioceptors between the atlas and occiput, the inner ear, and the position of the eyes in alignment with the horizon of the planet. As the client is seated in the chair looking out a window, or at a picture of nature on the wall, I will make very gentle contact with the client's chin and the back of his or her head.

Some clients have too much extension of their heads and others have too much flexion. The former appears to be looking up at the sky, however slightly, and the latter appears to be looking slightly down at the floor. The idea is to get the client's head properly placed on the neck so that the eyes are in alignment with the planet's horizon. Of course, practitioners will note such flexion or extension posture in clients and might work with the atlanto-occipital joint and related structures during the next session. Or it may be necessary to refer the client for soft-tissue work. But I have seen a few atlanto-occipital joints self-correct with horizon therapy, including my own.

Step 8: Now that the client has begun to breathe more functionally or appropriately and is aware of the accurate location of his or her head on the neck, I will begin working with the quality of attention. Horizon therapy is about toggling one's attention very slowly in the tempo of Primary Respiration from a focus on one's brain, eyes, and core of the body to a very unfocused attention out to nature. Nature here means the sky, the clouds, the sunshine, the trees, the wind, the squirrels on the fence, and so forth. The world of nature outside the window is the horizon, even if a visible horizon is not available. (When the visible horizon is available, such as at a beach, I encourage the client to practice there as well.)

I typically begin by asking clients to place their attention in the middle of their brain. I ask them to find the place between their nose and the back of the head. Sometimes I will even ask clients to roll their eyes up to the middle of their forehead for several seconds and then to relax their eyes. This puts a very slight tug on the third ventricle and is thus a good focus to sense the movement of Primary Respiration out to the horizon and back.

My job as practitioner is to verbally ask clients to move their attention slowly from focused to unfocused and back to focused on the brain and body as a whole. I am acting as a metronome, staying synchronized with my own Primary Respiration. This means that I ask clients to gaze out the window at nature, to defocus and relax their eyes. I guide them through the relaxation of all the muscles around their eyes and face, all the way down to their feet again. It is vital to perceive Primary Respiration by gently maintaining a sense of one's own three dimensionality at the same time as one is moving attention out to the horizon and back. I sometimes ask clients to look at their whole body as if their eyes were in the middle of their brain. Each client is different and different language may be needed to support the client—this is where the creativity of the practitioner is needed.

These steps and phases of horizon therapy need to be unfolded over several sessions. They cannot be given to clients all at once, but must be phased in little by little, session by session. Some practitioners actually like to teach this sequence of horizon therapy to their clients before a session even begins; I prefer the end, and it makes no difference. When clients feel comfortable with the practice, I may ask them during a session to periodically place their attention in the middle of their brain and take a deep breath, as indicated in step 4. This will further support the ignition process once the client is engaged in joint practice with the practitioner.

Step 9: Sometimes I put one hand on the front of the client's lower sternum and my back hand around the fifth thoracic vertebra. I ask the client to sense the movement of his or her heart. This is called interoceptive awareness or cardioception. When people can sustain attention on the movement of their own heart it has been shown to change the brain toward greater self-regulation. These are all skills that I teach my students and I adapt these practices for my clients. I remind the client that when he or she wakes up in the middle of the night it is very easy to sense the heart movement.

If clients cannot sense the heart movement with my hands on the front and back of the chest, I ask them to sense it in the middle of the night when they wake up and then to practice listening during the day. Gradually it is possible to sense the heart movements expand over more territory in the body three dimensionally. When heart movement awareness is combined with breath awareness, it is the best way to self-regulate stress. It is simply a matter of moving attention to the core of the body. When clients can sustain attention on their heart more easily, I ask them to say their favorite prayer silently in time with the beat of their heart. Most everyone has a favorite prayer or poem that they have memorized. This is also a great way to have a peaceful sleep.

Step 10: Finally, in order to fully engage clients and get their participation, I ask them to practice at home. I also know historically that most clients are overwhelmed with the nitty-gritty of their lives and simply don't do homework. So, when I give a client homework, it is from the point of view of being recommended, rather than required. I simply ask clients to sit on the edge of their bed when they get up in the morning or go to bed at night and look out a window and let their attention go. I try to help clients build in a conscious series of pauses in their daily routine, whether the pauses are the bookends of their day or simply a brief interlude in the middle of the day to look out a window and let the attention go out to the sky and the clouds. Attention is a lifestyle issue and an important health issue as well.

Over time, I may introduce clients to the term Primary Respiration, describing it as an approximately one-minute phase that moves the attention of the nervous system from inside the body out to nature and then a reverse phase for the same amount of time. All clients are capable of perceiving Primary Respiration. I have taught parents to perceive it in their children. Gradually clients can move from a fast tempo in their body to one in which they perceive the cycles of Primary Respiration and its dynamic relationship with stillness. A biodynamic session can continue all day and all night long.

The term *horizon therapy* was given to me by Katriona Forrester. Katriona was on a flight in Europe and was reading the airline magazine about a new European spa treatment called horizon therapy, in which people pay to go and sit outside and look at the horizon. Thank you, Katriona, for this insight into biodynamic practice.

I want to thank Tim Shafer for his excellent editorial suggestions, shaping a better way to help clients.

CHAPTER 12

Meditations on Ignition

Synchronizing Primary Respiration and Secondary Respiration

Primary Respiration generates secondary respiration.

1. The practitioner sits still and establishes three-dimensional buoyancy in her fluid body and orients to the central stillness.

   This is very similar to mindfulness meditation in the sense that the practitioner attends to the inhalation and exhalation of her biological breathing.

2. The practitioner begins to notice the brief gap of time between the inhalation and exhalation phase of secondary respiration. Then the practitioner begins to notice the brief gap at the end of the exhalation phase of secondary respiration before inhalation begins.

3. After several minutes of softening through the abdomen and rib cage and allowing biological breathing to inhale, gap, exhale, gap, the practitioner notices the end point of inhalation and observes if Primary Respiration is continuing to expand as the exhalation phase of secondary respiration begins. This is a subtle shift of attention into the three-dimensional fluid body.

4. The fulcrum for Primary Respiration is around the diaphragm. Thus the practitioner pays attention gently to the end point of her exhalation and notices if Primary Respiration continues to return in that phase of its breathing. Once contact is made with Primary Respiration, the practitioner toggles her attention back and forth from Primary to secondary respiration, exploring their unique relationship.

   Ignition points occur when the practitioner periodically takes a deep breath at the beginning of Primary Respiration expanding or returning.

An important component of this practice is to establish three dimensionality and a sense of the entire surface volume of the skin. This allows a sensibility to arise around the synchronization of Primary and secondary respiration.

Accessing the Third Ventricle

1. Sit in a comfortable meditative posture. Make sure the posture is not too rigid and not too loose. Do a body scan from the feet to the head and begin to sense the entire surface volume of the skin three dimensionally.

2. Gradually bring attention to the way the head is resting on the neck. Sense heaviness in the elbows and allow the shoulders to soften.

3. Bring attention to the occiput in the back of the head. Imagine the head is like a bobblehead doll and let more weight be experienced in the occiput in such a way that the head extends slightly with micro movement.

4. After a couple of minutes of sensing the occipital bobblehead, bring your attention around to the face and let the nose fall to gravity. This is the facial bobblehead doll.

5. After several minutes of experiencing the facial and occipital bobblehead, place attention directly in the space between the occiput and the face. This is generally in and around the third ventricle. Sense the central stillness from that place.

In order to assist the sensory acquisition of the third ventricle, it is helpful to close the eyes and allow the eyes to roll up to the middle of the forehead for several seconds and then relax the eyes. This puts a very slight tug on the anterior third ventricle via the optic chiasm.

Occasionally, the practitioner can roll her eyes up until it feels like it is easier to rest attention in the third ventricle. There may also be an ignition and permeation of potency releasing from the third ventricle when the eyes are rolled up to the middle of the forehead. It is very important to not hold the eyes in this position for more than several seconds at a time.

Gradually the practitioner combines these two practices—the synchronizing of the two breaths, above, and this one on the third ventricle. This is a powerful way for the practitioner to self-ignite during a session and help the client ignite.

Conclusion

When biodynamic work is correct, one's attention will naturally rest in the third ventricle, whether you are a practitioner or a client. In other words, I know as a client when a biodynamic practitioner is well bounded, I can access and rest in my third ventricle while receiving a session. Thus the ability to access and rest in the third ventricle is a barometer of the restorative function of biodynamic work with Primary Respiration.

I can also tell when a practitioner is too close because, as a client, if I try to access my third ventricle, I sometimes literally get bounced out of it. Then I have to let the practitioner know I need more space.

When meditation is coupled with sitting and looking at the horizon, it becomes a deeper form of an atlanto-occipital joint recalibration.

• • •

Photographic Text-Atlas of Biodynamic Skills

CHAPTER 13

Preliminary Instructions
and First Contact

How to View the Photographs

The intention of the photographs in this section is to provide a sense of precision for where the practitioner's hands are placed for any given location, or window, on the client's body. Precision is very important because the hands gradually change position naturally with micro movement and even periodically lift off the body due to the constant shaping of the fluid body. Thus the starting point is essential and there are many photographs that zoom in on my hands, not only on a skeleton, but also on my wife Cathy.

These photos span a period starting in 1990 and extending through the summer of 2010. The early photographs were taken during a time in my career when I was teaching biomechanical and functional approaches to craniosacral therapy. It has only been in the last decade that I have transitioned into the wholistic biodynamic approach. These photographs represent the complete way I practice and teach.

It is vitally important that the practitioner's arms and elbows have props such as a pillow or bolster underneath them during the use of certain positions. At no time should the practitioner's arms be suspended without a prop underneath them. As I say in class, the practitioner might need to stay steady for twenty minutes in one hand position, and it is difficult to predict when such a long time might be needed. The practitioner needs to have maximum comfort and ease, not only in each hand position, but also in one's posture during the entire length of every session. A good way to know this is by paying attention to one's breathing—if the practitioner's breathing is in any way restricted, the practitioner must change her posture to free the breathing.

Body alignment when seated, standing, or leaning over the client requires support and grounding for the whole body of the practitioner. One of the essential components of biodynamic practice is to maintain regular and almost vigilant contact with conscious somatic awareness. This is the essence of interpersonal neurobiology and, consequently, the foundation for empathy and the formation of compassionate responses that include knowing when to move one's hands to another location on the client. It is not necessary to look like a meditation expert with an upright posture whenever seated with hands on the client. I find myself frequently flexing my body forward, rolling my head or simply increasing or decreasing the lordosis in my lower back during a session while in contact with the client. In other words, it is okay to shift one's posture while hands are in contact with the client. Postural shifting needs to be done slowly and with micro movement.

It is necessary in the linear format of this book to divide the body into segments in order to present all the photographs. The sequence of the photographs as they are presented here is not necessarily a prescription or a protocol for practice. In general, I start my sessions either at the feet or in the Pietà position and try to sense the whole fluid body of the client breathing with Primary Respiration. Later in a session or subsequent session, I may address individual areas of interest in a client's body from the perspective of relating to the whole. The breathing whole is the most fundamental aspect of biodynamic practice. In addition, I rarely work on a client's head in the first several sessions. Likewise, I rarely do more than five or six hand positions in any given session.

That is the way I practice. The basic rule of thumb in the manual therapeutic arts is that one should never be a clone of one's teacher, but rather embody the work and own the work in order to keep it alive and fresh. Imitation is said to be the sincerest form of flattery and necessary at the beginning of the learning process. Then each practitioner must own the work for oneself. My suggestions are guidelines rather than statutory regulations. Find what works and discard the rest.

These photos and descriptions must only be used by practitioners with the training necessary for safe and effective practice. In no way are they intended for a beginner to practice without proper training and supervision.

Some photos only have brief references in the text and others have more detailed descriptions. As a convenience I have provided a brief description of all the photographs in Chapter 20. Some of the photo descriptions have an introduction in the following chapters. In the text I refer to hand positions as *windows*. Sometimes the hand positions are described in numbered *steps* because they take place in a sequence. Some windows are described as *variations*. Occasionally I provide more detail on the *process* involved with a particular window. Finally, I occasionally make a *summary* statement at the end of a window description.

The ground of biodynamic practice is covered in the following instructions and they apply to every hand position in this book. Periodically I repeat these basic instructions in the *process* paragraphs in the descriptions.

Preliminary Instructions Prior to Contact

Still Posture—Orienting

1. Biodynamic practice begins with the practitioner sitting still and upright with the knees slightly below the hips, feet flat on the ground, and head, neck, and shoulders in alignment. The posture is not too rigid and not too loose. I like to imagine my umbilicus, heart, and third ventricle all lined up as I sit in preparation.

2. The practitioner begins attending to her respiratory diaphragm, gradually breathing into her entire soma from head to foot as if filling up and deflating a living skin balloon. Being aware of thinking and slowing down the stream of mental thoughts by shifting attention to breathing is essential. Whenever the wandering mind goes off (and it will), simply and gently bring attention back to breathing.

   The intention is to become self aware and to find the mind of equanimity and serenity and to establish a three-dimensional (3D) sense of the environment surrounding the practitioner's fluid body. This starts by sensing the total surface of the skin from the outside and the inside. The practitioner maintains an orientation to present time with the location of attention slowly switching between breathing, one's body, and its shape determined by the skin and the environment (the zones). See Chapter 5.

This begins the practitioner's slowing and stilling process with which the client resonates through the interpersonal brain and heart systems. It establishes an embodied sense of empathy, insight, and compassion.

I like to tell the client at the beginning of a session that I am going to take a couple of minutes to settle myself. I take that time to practice these first few steps of orienting, synchronizing, and attuning to establish attention in present time.

Three-Dimensional Fluid Body—Spinal Synchronization

1. The next phase is for the practitioner to sense and image her body as a three-dimensional (3D), transparent, living fluid continuum. First, she senses the total surface volume of the skin, which establishes an orientation to her fluid

body as a single shape. The fluid body can be sensed under the skin as an ocean within and all over the surface of the skin as if being contained in an egg-shaped vessel, just as it was in the embryo being surrounded by an amniotic sac and a chorionic sac.

2. For healing to happen, both the practitioner and the client symbolically return to the undifferentiated wholeness of the original fluid body in the early embryo. This state is available in present time through the courtesy of Primary Respiration. In other words, the historical and contemporary trauma story is replaced with the origin story of love via the perception of Primary Respiration (PR) and stillness in present time through the medium of the fluid body.

3. The practitioner then begins to sense PR moving up and down the middle of her spine like an accordion lengthening and shortening every fifty seconds. The spine is imaged as a tube suspended inside the 3D fluid body. Alternatively, the practitioner may sense Primary Respiration moving three dimensionally out and back from around the respiratory diaphragm.

Heart Mirror and Third Ventricle Synchronization

1. The practitioner then imagines the space of her hands, arms, and trunk as one big heart mirror rounded like a satellite dish and extending from side to side in the trunk and abdomen and from top to bottom from the nose down to the pubic bone.

   The intention is to perceive PR coming from the client with the sternum and heart area of the practitioner rather than with the hands initially. The practitioner is sitting at the side or feet of the client using the heart mirror.

2. PR moves beyond the surface of the skin and can be felt through attention on the heart, umbilicus, or third ventricle (3V). This means that the practitioner might also sense PR moving from her 3V out to the horizon and back and then between her heart and the heart of the client. In order to bring attention to the 3V, I recommend closing the eyes and rolling the eyes up and in toward the middle of the forehead for several seconds and then relaxing the eyes. This makes it a little easier to rest attention in the third ventricle.

This begins the process of becoming receptive and yielding to the flow of PR and stillness coming from the client and/or the horizon once contact is made. During a session, the practitioner toggles back and forth from her umbilicus to her heart to her third ventricle or to her spine in order to sense PR. Usually one or the other location is prominent in any given session so it is important to practice with all four locations to locate the most readily available access point of PR at a given time. Every session is different.

It is vitally important to sit and sense the literal movement of the heart inside one's trunk as frequently as possible in a session and between sessions.

First Touch

1. The practitioner sits by the side of the client's body to practice the Pietà window (described below). Each hand position on the client is called a *window*. It is a window of observing the activity of the fluid body at its surface. There is no intention or effort to look below the surface of the skin for biodynamic practice. Many practitioners have previous training in models of work that look inside the client's body. That has its place once the fluid body has stabilized and begun to breathe with Primary Respiration and only in small increments. This means for only several seconds or minutes in the middle of a session and only if the practitioner knows how to balance the fluid body if it has withdrawn or become compressed as a result. Everything necessary for the practitioner to know and perceive floats to the surface under the guidance of PR.

2. The practitioner verbally asks permission to make contact after sensing PR in the client with the heart mirror mentioned above. This verbal permission is usually done at least once and always at the beginning of a session.

3. Upon contact, the practitioner immediately becomes receptive and reorients and resynchronizes with her own heart and fluid body. This means removing her attention from her hands for a brief period of time in order to establish the therapeutic relationship as a circulatory system or a two-person biology. This is the cycle of attunement. The client needs to orient to the practitioner's nervous and circulatory systems first.

4. To develop afferent or sensory touch in the hands, the practitioner periodically maintains attention at the back of her hands and body while in contact with the client. The practitioner's body and hands are buoyant and transparent like a cork floating in water.

5. The initial therapeutic exploration is to sense the entire fluid body of the client as a single whole continuum breathing at the rate of PR. This is done *after* the practitioner senses her own fluid body breathing with PR.

This gives the client the space to feel safety and trust in the relationship. All normal change from a biodynamic point of view is oriented to stillness and PR.

Biodynamic palpation involves sensing systemic shape changes in the client's fluid body rather than tissue changes, although they are related. The question to be explored is whether the client's fluid body has a stronger or more amplified ability to breathe with PR at the end of a session. Consequently, its capacity to breathe with PR must be assessed at the beginning if a session.

Pietà

1. The client is supine. The practitioner sits at the side of the client with the practitioner's body perpendicular to the client opposite the client's heart and diaphragm. One hand is placed palm up under the upper arm and shoulder of the client while the opposite hand is palm up under the leg of the client, approximately under the knee depending on the arm length of the practitioner, as if holding a bowl of living water. See Figures 13.1 and 13.2.

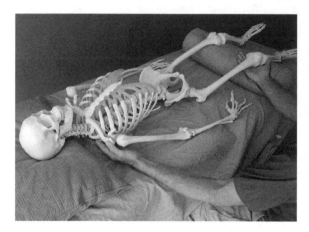

Figure 13.1. Pietà a

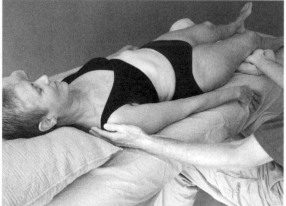

Figure 13.2. Pietà b

2. Practice a cycle of attunement, detailed below. The practitioner comes into relationship with the client with the heart dish, then her hands, then back to herself, synchronizing with PR while slowly moving her attention to and from the horizon. This establishes evenly suspended attention.

3. Practitioner images wholeness and eggness as a 3D reality in present time in and around her hands, her body, and that of the client. Primary Respiration is the living movement of wholeness.

Feet

1. The client is supine. The practitioner is sitting in alignment with the spinal midline of the client at the feet. This notochordal midline in the spine shortens during inhalation and lengthens during exhalation of PR as mentioned above

in the spinal accordion perception. The practitioner practices the heart mirror to sense being moved by PR from the client's midline.

2. Then the practitioner contacts the dorsum of the feet bilaterally, or alternatively holds the heels in the palms of her hands (Figure 13.3). She reorients, resynchronizes, and practices a cycle of attunement.

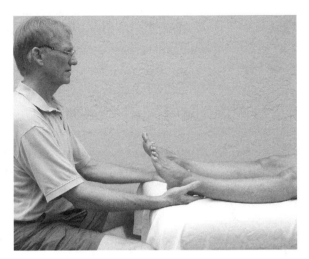

Figure 13.3. Feet

3. The practitioner periodically visualizes the whole transparent fluid body in the client when she brings her attention to her hands while synchronizing with PR. This visualizing practice can happen in each window, but only for several seconds. It is important to sense whether the fluid body of the client contracts or expands with the visualization. If it contracts then it is contraindicated to visualize the client in that way at that time. The practitioner can focus on visualizing her own fluid body or go to the horizon and back with PR.

This window helps to thaw out the fight-flight response that has imploded in the interosseous membrane between the tibia and fibula. It lowers autonomic tone.

Cycle of Attunement

1. Attunement, the movement of attention, is practiced in each window. A *cycle of attunement* is the basic unit of perceptual work in a biodynamic session. This bears repeating:

    The practitioner moves her attention toward her hands and away from her hands at the tempo of PR and then expands into the stillness from one of her fulcrums such as the umbilicus, heart, or third ventricle out to the horizon (zone D) and back at the tempo of PR. This cycle of attunement is repeated periodically during a session.

2. Gradually the practitioner's attention becomes suspended between a fulcrum, especially the third ventricle, and the horizon so that very little effort is needed to move attention between those locations.

Different tempos establish structure and function in the shape of the embryo. The tempo of PR is the essential catalytic factor that modifies and generates order and organization throughout the life span. This means that it tempers the speed and heat generated by compressive and rapid cellular forces moving in the embryo. PR provides order and organization for growth and development. Such order and/or organization is oriented to the symmetry of the initial embryonic fulcrums that become the umbilicus, heart, and third ventricle. This is why the practitioner orients to such in herself during a session.

Practitioner attunement normalizes imprinting from the preverbal time of life. This also includes the infant-mother attachment process and consequently the adult therapeutic relationship. The goal is for the practitioner to build self-regulation and integration in herself, which creates resonance for the client's nervous system to orient to and thus may stabilize the client's nervous system.

CHAPTER 14

Lower Extremities

Lower Extremities Supine

1. The client is supine. Practitioner is seated at the end of the table. Starting with either foot, contact each foot of the client individually with index finger and thumb of both hands holding the cuboid-navicular bone relationship. The index fingers are on the top surface of the client's foot and thumbs are below (Figures 14.1 and 14.2). It has been said in osteopathy that the cuboid-navicular relationship is analogous to the sphenoid-occiput relationship and that there is a fascial connection between the two.

   The practitioner's hands look like they are playing a flute while on the client's foot. The middle fingers or index fingers are touching together on the dorsum of one of the client's feet.

   The precise contact with the pads of these fingers is one on top of the cuboid bone and the other on top of the navicular bone. The thumb tips are

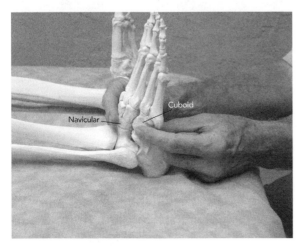

Figure 14.1. Cuboid-navicular a

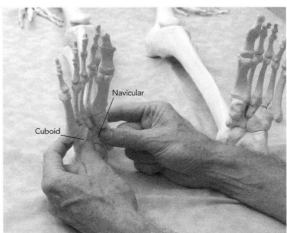

Figure 14.2. Cuboid-navicular b

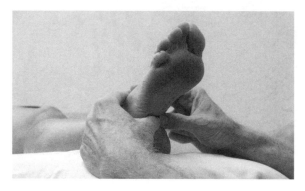

Figure 14.3. Cuboid-navicular c

touching below directly underneath the cuboid and navicular bones. See Figure 14.3.

The practitioner waits for Primary Respiration (PR) to breathe the bones until they remold or relax.

Each foot can be done or just one.

2. The next sequence for the lower extremity is also with the client supine. From the side of the table, the practitioner cradles the ankle with one hand in order to contact the medial and lateral malleoli. The other hand of the practitioner is cupping the posterior-inferior popliteal space of the knee. See Figures 14.4, 14.5, and 14.6.

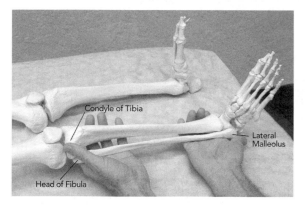

Figure 14.4. Legs supine a

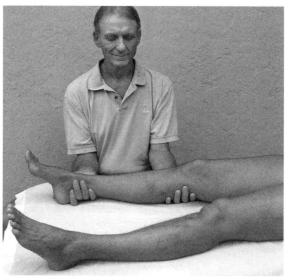

Figure 14.5. Legs supine b

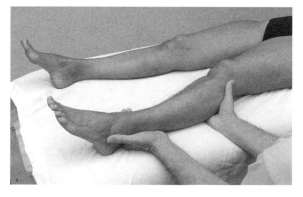

Figure 14.6. Legs supine c

Depending on the size of the practitioner's hands, the hand under the knee can be in contact with the head of the fibula and part of the tibial plateau. This is a noncranium vault hold in order to sense PR breathing the lower extremity through the interosseous membrane.

It is here where imploded fight-flight energy can become imprinted. This is an excellent way to stabilize the ANS.

3. Once the practitioner senses PR in the lower extremity, she switches hands so the bottom hand moves from the ankle to the knee while the top hand moves to contact with the fifth lumbar vertebra (L5). L5 is the osseous fulcrum for the lower extremity. The practitioner waits to sense Primary Respiration breathing between her two hands. See Figures 14.7 and 14.8.

Sometimes in a client with a lot of low back, pelvic, and/or extremity issues, the osseous fulcrum can shift higher up in the lumbars or lower down in the sacrum. The practitioner may need to shift her hands slightly to find the fulcrum location.

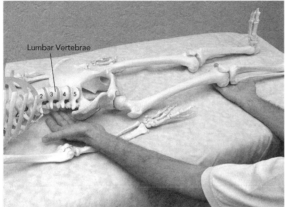

Figure 14.7. Legs supine d

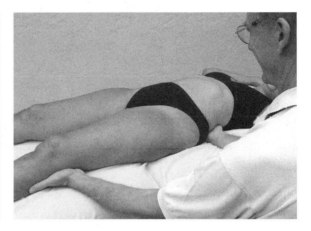

Figure 14.8. Legs supine e

Lower Extremities in Sidelying

1. Practitioner starts with the cuboid-navicular window, as in the previous sequence, with the client supine (illustrated in Figures 14.1, 14.2, and 14.3). The subsequent hand positions are done with the client in sidelying.

2. The client is sidelying with the knees and feet stacked evenly upon each other and the knees slightly flexed.

The practitioner makes contact with the head of the fibula and the lateral malleoli. The practitioner's index finger and thumb are together as if plucking a tissue out of a box of Kleenex. This style of contact is used with both hands on the proximal and distal ends of the fibula of the client. See Figures 14.9, 14.10, and 14.11.

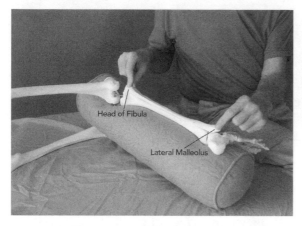

Figure 14.9. Lower extremity in sidelying a

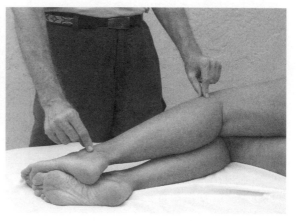

Figure 14.10. Lower extremity in sidelying b

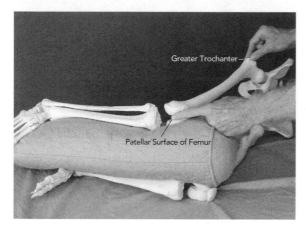

Figure 14.11. Lower extremity in sidelying c

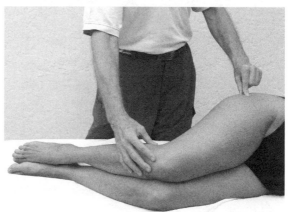

Figure 14.12. Lower extremity in sidelying d

The practitioner waits until PR begins to breathe the intraosseous fibula. Other motions especially lengthening may occur until the bone softens and becomes flexible.

3. The client is sidelying with the knees and feet stacked evenly upon each other and the knees slightly flexed.

The practitioner makes contact with the greater trochanter and the space between the patella and tibial plateau. See Figure 14.12. The finger contact with the trochanter is the same as above in the tissue-plucking position; however, the other hand of the practitioner is simply using the pads of one or two fingers in the space between the patella and tibial plateau in order to be relatively close to the distal end of the femur.

As above, the practitioner waits for the femur to begin breathing with PR.

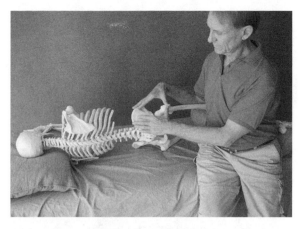

Figure 14.13. Lower extremity in sidelying e

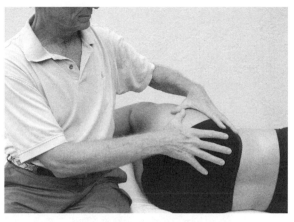

Figure 14.14. Lower extremity in sidelying f

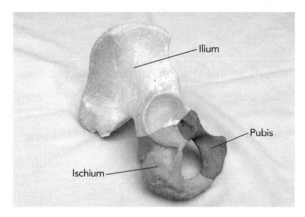

Figure 14.15. Embryological derivatives
of the innominate bone

4. The client is sidelying with the knees and feet stacked evenly upon each other and the knees slightly flexed.

   The practitioner crosses her thumbs and imagines that her hands are like the wings of a bird. See Figures 14.13 and 14.14.

   The thumbs are placed over the greater trochanter of the client's hip. The practitioner's fingers spread out and span from the crest of the ilium anteriorly to the anterior superior iliac spine.

   PR will begin to breathe the three embryological derivatives of the innominate bones: the ischium, the ilium, and the pubic bone. Their fulcrum is in the acetabular fossa. See Figure 14.15. There is also a transverse midline between the two acetabular fossae that may manifest and begin to breathe with PR.

   Wait for nutation and counternutation of the innominates to normalize.

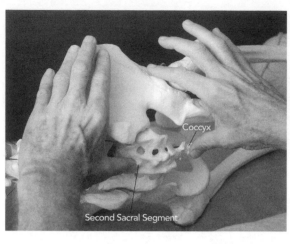

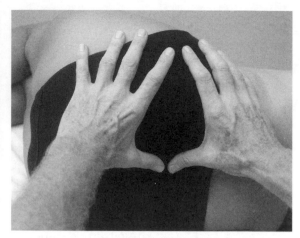

Figure 14.16. Lower extremity in sidelying g

Figure 14.17. Lower extremity in sidelying h

5. The client is sidelying with the knees and feet stacked evenly upon each other and the knees slightly flexed.

The practitioner places the pad of one thumb on the sacral base and the pad of the opposite thumb around or near the coccyx of the client. See Figures 14.16 and 14.17.

Wait for the sacrum to breathe with PR and normalize its motion with the spine and innominates.

CHAPTER 15

Abdomen and Pelvis

Developmental Movements of the Midgut

As the endoderm develops into a definitive tube by about the fourth week post-fertilization, it is divided into three distinct areas. The foregut is very large and wide and makes up all the structures or most of the face and neck because of the pharyngeal arches. This includes the esophagus, the stomach, the liver, the gall bladder, the lungs, and the pancreas. These are derived from the foregut, where the tube is the biggest and widest.

The midgut is attached to the yolk sac by means of the vitelline artery and vein. The mesenteries, the small intestine, and large intestine derive from the midgut in relationship to a substantial shaping process oriented to the superior mesenteric artery and the yolk sac.

The hindgut is slow growing and consists of the urogenital system and those respective organs. The hindgut is attached to the bony pelvis and as such is anchored to the sacrum. Consequently, both the foregut and hindgut have a hard covering around them, so to speak. That is the facial bones and pelvic bones.

For the sake of this exploration, the practitioner first must differentiate between metabolic movements involving the slow tempo of Primary Respiration (PR), then if possible the physiological and cardiovascular movements coming from the tempos in the Mid Tide, and finally the motility from the final adult form of the organ. Motility, which is a faster tempo, describes the motion present in an organ as it is held in its fascial container in relationship to adjacent structures.

1. The client is supine. Figure 15.1 shows the geography of the abdomen. It is not necessary to have skin-to-skin contact with the client by the practitioner's hands. I recommend that the practitioner sit at the side of the table with proper support for the arms and elbows. In this way, the hands are placed

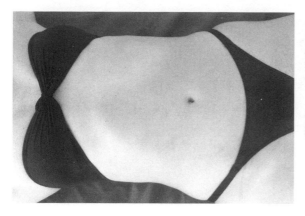

Figure 15.1. Umbilicus a

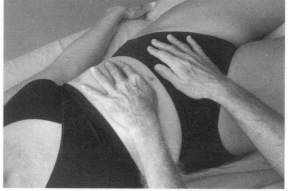

Figure 15.2. Umbilicus b

palm down above and below the umbilicus of the client, but not over the top of the client's umbilicus, as in Figure 15.2.

The first exploration is tuning in to the superior mesenteric artery. This artery originally was directly posterior to the umbilicus and it grows from posterior to anterior toward the umbilicus to innervate the intestines. Consequently, the superior mesenteric artery could be considered a horizontal midline for the development of the midgut.

The developing intestines at four weeks postfertilization begin to herniate out of the umbilicus and into the yolk sac. This is a posterior-to-anterior movement through the fulcrum of the umbilicus and caused by a differential in the coelomic space available, which is next to none in the embryo, in order to accommodate the fast-growing intestines. Consequently, they must grow out of the body initially.

In order to grow out, the intestines do it in a spiral motion following the growth of the superior mesenteric artery. This is a 90-degree counterclockwise motion around the umbilicus.

2. Next, there is a three-dimensional expansion of the intestines in all directions. This is related to a dilation field.

3. Following that, there is a retraction of the intestines toward the spine as more space becomes available in the coelomic cavity or core of the developing embryo. At this point in development, consider that the coelomic cavity is expanding and there are significant growth movements going inferiorly toward the hindgut and superiorly toward the brain. These growth movements and space are pulling the intestines back into place within the coelomic cavity. The practitioner needs to think and perceive three dimensionally.

As the intestines retract toward the posterior abdominal wall, they do so in a continuing spiral which is a 180-degree counterclockwise motion.

This spiral motion is a result of the movement of the blood in the superior mesenteric artery. Consequently, it is important to stay attuned to this artery when working around the umbilicus.

4. Next, the intestines start to develop shearing motions three dimensionally because of the differential sizes of the small and large intestines. There may also be transverse motions and other vectors because of the rapid growth and compression of the intestines into the abdominal space. In other words, the intestines are getting compacted.

   Consequently, there will also be a strong sense of compression at this phase of development. This compression can be very similar and actually mimic the compression from the first week postfertilization.

5. During the next phase, there will be a three-dimensional expansion with a particular emphasis on an inferior vector funneling down toward the anus and coccyx. This, of course, will be the descending colon and rectum. This expansion downward toward the coccyx is done in conjunction with the growth of the genitals and the kidney-bladder system.

   At about eleven weeks, there will be a fusion of the mesenteries up against the posterior abdominal wall with condensation of the intestines as the embryo transitions into the fetal period of life. The attachment of the mesentery to the posterior abdominal wall is on a line from the ileocecal valve to the duojejunal junction. This is a diagonal line and the abdominal aorta lies right on top of it.

6. Finally, there is a very significant channel of potency moving in and out of the umbilicus. It is differentiated into both vitelline circulation coming from the yolk sac and placental circulation coming from the connecting stalk that contains the umbilical veins and arteries. Remember that Primary Respiration (PR) as it comes through the umbilical cord is associated with the quality of loving kindness.

Process: Periodically in these steps the practitioner may imagine a yolk sac as a dome over the entire ventral (front) surface of the client's body. Likewise, the amniotic sac can be imaged as a fluid-filled dome under the entire dorsal (back) surface of the client's body. Anytime the practitioner visualizes a fluid sphere around or in the client, she must be able to distinguish if the fluid body of the client expands or contracts as a reaction to the visualization. If the fluid body contracts then the visualization is contraindicated.

Summary: It must be remembered that the development of the gut tube is intimately related to the development of the cardiovascular system. Embryonic blood is produced in the yolk sac and circulates back into the embryo via the vitelline artery and vein. The celiac artery, the superior mesenteric artery, and inferior mesenteric artery are the three major fulcrums for the midgut and lower part of the foregut and upper part of the hindgut.

First Gaze—Umbilical Cord Supine

This exploration takes into account a sequence of events spanning fetal placental development all the way up to a sequence of events immediately following birth. In general, it comes from a set of skills related to birth ignition. Birth ignition takes into account a sequence of events as mentioned in my Volume Two, immediately after the infant's body is fully out of the birth canal and has taken its first breath. The optimal sequence is:

- The first skin-to-skin contact with the mother, usually on the mother's abdomen and chest, which is called sustained skin contact (SSC), necessary to establish thermal regulation (heat distribution) and ignite the capacities of digestion, absorption, and elimination from breastfeeding
- The infant crawling up the mother's abdomen and chest to begin breastfeeding
- The first gaze of the mother at her newborn on her breast
- The first gaze of the infant at her mother's eyes from the position of the mother's breast (This mutual gazing, in conjunction with breastfeeding and sustained skin contact, allows unconditional love to be given, received, and embodied by the infant.)
- Cutting the umbilical cord
- The birth and death of the placenta

Window: This window involves the client being in supine position with a bolster under his knees. The practitioner will also need to have props for the elbows and arms, because she will place both hands palm down on the client's abdomen. The practitioner's touch is very buoyant and focused on the backs of the hands.

The practitioner is sensing the client from the back of her hands, arms, and body. If at all possible, the practitioner's hands should be able to have skin-to-skin contact with the client's abdomen. It has been my experience that some clients are very uncomfortable having their abdomen touched. In some cases, I've actually placed a towel over the client's shirt for extra covering over the abdomen.

Permission for such skin-to-skin contact must be negotiated prior to making the contact itself. The client needs to be informed that skin-to-skin contact is preferable with this window before the session starts.

Process: The skill involved with this window has several extra elements associated with it. First, the practitioner considers her arms and hands to be the umbilical cord in the position shown in Figure 15.2. It is very helpful to develop a three-dimensional sense of the movement and activity of the practitioner's heart, including a pulsation down through the arms into the hands. Frequently, as the practitioner deepens into this skill, she will sense a pulsation where the hands are making contact with the client's abdomen. This indeed is the pulsation of the umbilical cord itself as two mutually interacting cardiovascular systems are speaking with each other heart to heart.

The next skill involves the practitioner visualizing herself as the mother of the client and the client as the placenta. In other words, she visualizes the entire body of the client as this gorgeous, pulsing, blood-filled, living placenta. Recent research in fetal placental development has shown that the human placenta has its own nervous system, endocrine system, immune system, and cardiovascular system. The placenta could almost be considered the fetal twin. It is 25 percent of the fetal-placental relationship by volume. This is a good reminder that the placenta should no longer be considered merely a filtration system. It is an active unique body and a vital part of our early somatic reality that dies at birth.

Periodically, in the cycle of attunement process, as the practitioner moves her attention out and back from the natural world, she will trade places with the client imaginally and become the placenta. Thus the client will then become the mother person. This role reversal is a critical part of this biodynamic skill and many others. The question becomes when is this window finished and how does the practitioner discern a change? When stillness permeates the room and the client's body or when Primary Respiration (PR) increases its potency or amplitude is when the practitioner can move on or finish the session.

Finally, the practitioner occasionally looks at the client's face and has a smile of loving kindness just as if the practitioner as mother was looking at her baby for the very first time after birth. This is called the first gaze. Likewise, when the practitioner places her hands on the client's abdomen, this can be equated with the first touch, as mentioned above. Together with the first breath, described in Volume Two, the first gaze and the first touch when coupled with PR are able to begin to normalize the harm of birth-related stress and trauma.

Umbilical Cord Prone

This particular window is designed to give the practitioner easy access to three biodynamic properties. The first is that of the fluid body. The second is that of the embryological derivatives of the midgut from the stomach to the distal end of the large intestine. Finally, the third part of this skill is balancing and restorative for the interrelationship of the respiratory diaphragm to the pelvic diaphragm.

Window: The client is in prone position, seen in Figure 15.3. If possible, the client's head needs to be supported by a face cradle inserted into the end of the treatment table. A bolster should be placed under the client's ankles. Some clients will not be able to lie prone on the table, especially during pregnancy; this position is contraindicated for these clients.

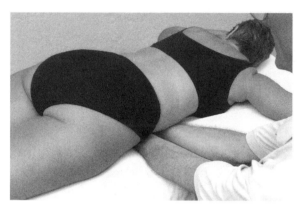

Figure 15.3. Umbilicus c

After orienting, synchronizing, and attuning, the practitioner observes the quality and three dimensionality of the client's secondary respiration. For example, when the client breathes in, does the movement of the respiratory diaphragm translate into movement of the sacrum? The next step is to negotiate permission to make contact. *Both of the practitioner's hands are palm up and go directly underneath the client's abdomen directly around the umbilicus.* The hands can cross the midline with one hand above the umbilicus and the other hand below the umbilicus. Every attempt should be made to avoid contact with the pubic symphysis and/or the xyphoid process and medial aspect of the costal arch. In other words, do not allow the hands to cover the umbilicus of the client. If at all possible, the practitioner's hands should be able to have skin-to-skin contact with the client's abdomen. The client needs to be informed that skin-to-skin contact is preferable with this window before the session begins.

Process: Now the practitioner can reorient, resynchronize, and reattune. When the practitioner attends to her hands, it is for the purpose of exploring the above intentions. The first intention is to sense the fluid body breathing three dimensionally with PR. The second intention is to notice any of the developmental movements of the midgut, discussed at the beginning of this chapter.

Summary: This skill gives the practitioner the ability to observe a new state of balance between the respiratory diaphragm and the pelvic diaphragm. These two diaphragms are designed to move reciprocally. They are interconnected via several layers of fascia. Typically, the practitioner only has to observe the movement and activity of the client's respiration because it is the strongest sensation and movement that the hands can feel in this location. Consequently, just the hand position itself is an invitation for these two diaphragms to balance themselves together. Gradually, the practitioner will be able to sense how the client's breathing moves down into the pelvis and there will be an ignition as both diaphragms synchronize their activity.

Many clients have had surgeries affecting their pelvic floor organs, such as hysterectomies, prostatectomies, or colon resectioning. All such surgical interventions on the pelvic floor and the midgut will create adhesions in the fascial and diaphragmatic system, translating into a loss of motion and function. Such losses can also occur from food allergies and inflammatory conditions in the gut, as discussed in Chapters 1 through 4. In these cases, coming into relationship with the sacrum, as well as more specific windows around the respiratory diaphragm, will be invaluable.

Primitive Streak—Sacrum Supine

Window: Figure 15.4 shows the basic geography of the sacrum while the client is prone. Figure 15.5 shows how to palpate the sacrum with the client prone. If the new practitioner is not familiar with the sacrum, I recommend beginning to palpate it with the client prone.

Practitioner is seated perpendicular to the client. The client is supine. One hand is contacting the sacral base and the spinous processes of the fourth and fifth lumbar vertebrae (L4–L5), as shown in Figures 15.6 and 15.7. The third finger (or longest finger or most comfortable finger) of the other hand contacts the coccyx gently and then relaxes slightly off of the coccyx. The practitioner *does not lift* the sacrum. She approaches from the side under the client's leg by the gluteal fold with the bottom hand and above the crest of the ilium with the other hand, as shown in Figure 15.8. She then reorients, resynchronizes, and completes a cycle of attunement.

The practitioner may sense the space all around and in the sacrum breathe and come alive with PR, like a flower opening and closing. Other possibilities include sensing a longitudinal fluctuation of the fluid body like an electric current going up to the client's head and the movement of the neural tube itself. (The longitudinal fluctuation is discussed at length at the end of this chapter.) It is important for the practitioner to stay three-dimensional (3D). The practitioner then completes several cycles of attunement.

Summary: The primitive streak is crucial for embodiment, for creation of the whole pelvis, and for generation of the heart. It induces cells to form the cardiovascular and musculoskeletal systems. It initiates the formation of the

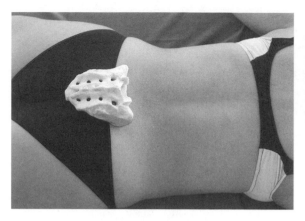

Figure 15.4. Sacrum a

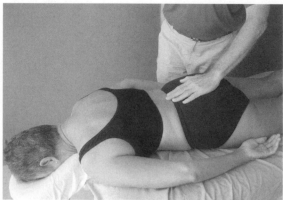

Figure 15.5. Sacrum b

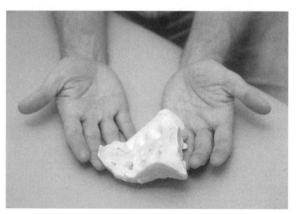

Figure 15.6. Sacrum c

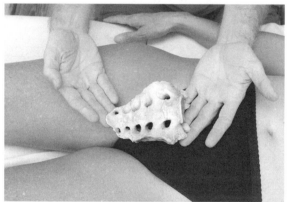

Figure 15.7. Sacrum d

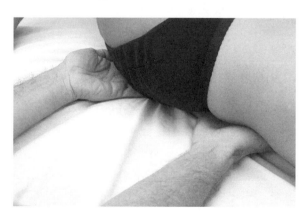

Figure 15.8. Sacrum e

notochord, which is related to the spine and cranial base.

This window also helps to normalize the autonomic nervous system (ANS) of the client. This means that the ANS needs to have a relative amount of disengagement from high or low tone in order for PR to express its healing priorities and allow the client to become conscious of its activity and subtlety. This event was called "idling" by Dr. Sutherland. The ANS will idle and PR will move the fluid body into deeper balance. The most important instruction for the practitioner is to wait patiently.

Liver

The liver is an extremely important organ in core regulation. As food breaks down in the intestines, it passes through the villi into the bloodstream. All of the digested and undigested food goes into the portal vein and is carried to the liver for processing. Embryologically, the liver forms the outer layer of the developing heart and itself begins as an engorgement of blood vessels. Treating the liver is a good way to explore the heart.

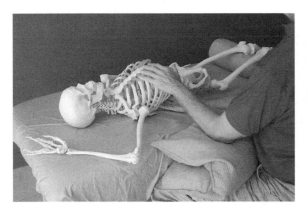

Figure15.9. Liver a

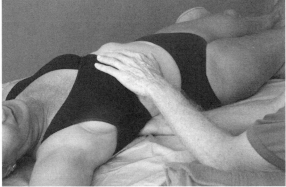

Figure 15.10. Liver b

Window: The client is supine and the practitioner's hands are surrounding the liver from the right side of the client, as shown in Figures 15.9, 15.10, and 15.11. Typically the left hand of the practitioner is under ribs 7–10 and the top hand is above the costal arch with the little finger and hypothenar eminence straddling the costal arch. It is important to have good support under the right arm and elbow in order to make buoyant contact with the client's rib cage.

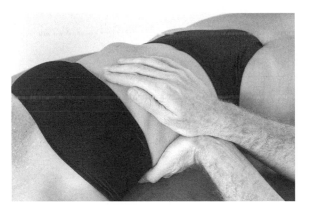

Figure 15.11. Liver c

Process: The practitioner begins to ride the rise and fall of the client's rib cage as he is breathing. The hands simply are a cork floating on this movement.

Gradually, a deeper awareness of the liver rises to the surface above the diaphragmatic movement. The practitioner is listening for PR from the embryological vector of the liver's origin from the midgut, which would now be the juncture of approximately where the esophagus passes through the diaphragm.

The practitioner settles into a relationship with PR in the client's liver while practicing several cycles of attunement. The practitioner may encounter a very deep stillness in the liver and the possibility of this stillness expanding out to zone D.

Bladder

The bladder forms from the fourth fluid cavity in the embryo called the allantois. The other three cavities are yolk, amnion, and chorion. The allantois protrudes into the developing connecting stalk, soon to be the umbilical cord. Some embryologists say that the allantois induces the umbilical veins and arteries to form.

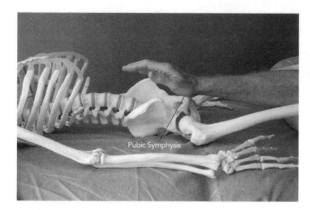

Figure 15.12. Bladder a

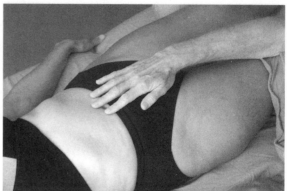

Figure 15.13. Bladder b

Window: The client is supine. Sometimes it might help to ask the client to move his body a little closer to the edge of the table depending on the hand dominance of the practitioner. The practitioner sits on the edge of the table or stands and asks the client to point out the location of his pubic symphysis. Then the practitioner places the heel of her dominant or preferred hand on top of the pubic symphysis, with the fingers on the abdomen pointing toward the umbilicus, as shown in Figures 15.12 and 15.13.

The practitioner imagines the original allantois as a fluid-filled cavity (the bladder in this case) that comes up, around, and on top of the pubic symphysis. While attuning to PR in the bladder, the practitioner's hands have a tendency to rock forward in an arc and then back rhythmically with PR.

Once the practitioner is familiar with this hand position and the movement of the bladder with PR, she can sit at the side of the client in a chair and use the hypothenar eminence (base of the small finger) of her hand to contact the pubic symphysis. The thumb is pointing toward the umbilicus. This helps balance the support ligaments of the bladder that go up to the umbilicus.

Alternatively, the opposite hand can be placed over the costal arch (over the liver) in order to balance the bladder and liver together.

Summary: The bladder is the main support organ of the pelvic floor, with very strong attachments to the posterior border of the pubic symphysis. The prostate, uterus, and cervix are suspended from the bladder and the sacrum. This is a very important organ that facilitates core regulation in the hindgut or pelvic floor.

Small Intestine

The small intestine develops in the embryo by spiraling out of the coelomic sac (abdominal area) along with the mesenteric artery. The small intestine and large intestine actually grow into the vitelline duct and yolk sac.

Window: The client is supine and, as with the bladder, both hands are placed immediately around the umbilicus with the fingers pointing toward the rib cage, as shown in Figure 15.14. Recall that PR moves in a spiral.

Process: Sometimes the hands of the practitioner may feel like they are being lifted off of the body and brought back down. Sometimes the hands simply stay in buoyant contact.

As with the bladder, once the practitioner is familiar with this movement, she may sit at the side and place the hands perpendicular to the body above and below the umbilicus.

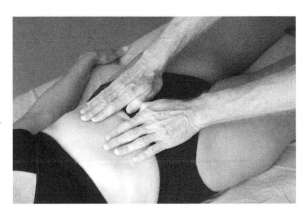

Figure 15.14. Small intestine

Large Intestine

The large intestine has the same developmental vector as the small intestine. I like to differentiate these two structures in the adult because of the different challenges that infants, children, adolescents, and adults face with their small intestine and large intestine. This includes everything from gluten sensitivity to constipation and complex inflammatory processes, as discussed in Chapters 1 through 4.

Window: The client is supine and, just as was done with the bladder and small intestine, the practitioner sits on the edge of the table and places her hands as laterally as possible on the belly, equidistant from the umbilicus, as shown in Figure 15.15. Sitting on the right side of the client, the practitioner's left hand

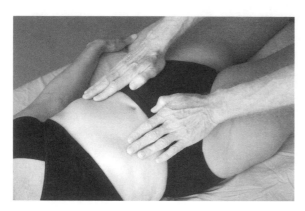

Figure 15.15. Large intestine

will be over the ascending colon of the client. The ascending colon is on the surface of the abdomen.

Process: The basic movement is that of a spiral, as noted above for the small intestine when exploring with PR. The main challenge with this window is that it is difficult to do while sitting perpendicular to the client (at the side).

The practitioner should solicit verbally any signs or signals of discomfort that the client might be having.

Summary: When exploring with these viscera in a biodynamic session, only two organs should be explored during any one session.

The Pelvic and Respiratory Diaphragms

Window: Client is supine with the practitioner sitting at the client's pelvis.

Practitioner orients, synchronizes, and attunes. She places one hand under the coccyx and waits. She places the other hand under the respiratory diaphragm. She allows the two diaphragms to synchronize their motion with PR.

The practitioner places both hands under the respiratory diaphragm from the side and imagines there is no respiratory diaphragm present, only one fluid cavity (see Figures 15.16 and 15.17). This balances the heart, the abdomen, and the pelvic floor.

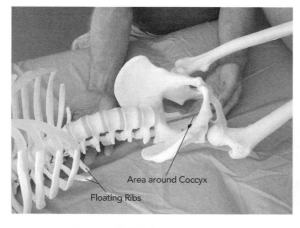

Area around Coccyx

Floating Ribs

Figure 15.16. Diaphragms a

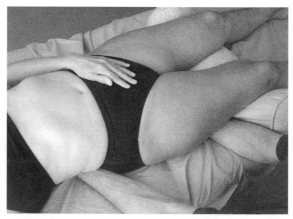

Figure 15.17. Diaphragms b

Kidneys Prone

Window: The client is prone, with head supported in a head rest if possible. The practitioner's hands are on the kidneys bilaterally, as shown in Figure 15.18. It is important to discover how the kidneys move with PR. The embryonic kidneys go all the way up to the neck and the adult kidneys expand and contract with PR on a vector toward the heart and away from the heart.

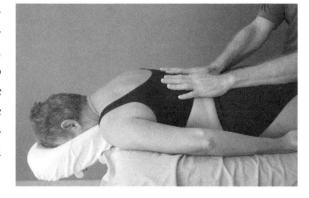

Figure 15.18. Kidneys

Hip Bones Supine

Window: Practitioner's hands are supporting the entire hip bone, as shown in Figure 15.19. The top hand has contact with the anterior superior iliac spine. The bottom hand has contact with the ischial tuberosity. The fingers do not need to be under the tuberosity, but merely touching it from the side.

Sometimes, the client needs to be asked to lift up the hip so the practitioner can make contact with the tuberosity underneath, as shown in Figure 15.20. Then instruct the client to relax the hip on top of the hand, as shown in Figure 15.21.

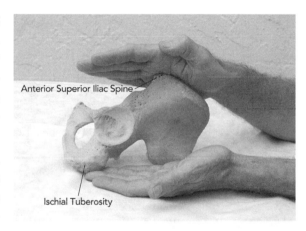

Figure 15.19. Hip bones supine a

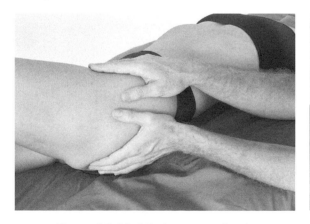

Figure 15.20. Hip bones supine b

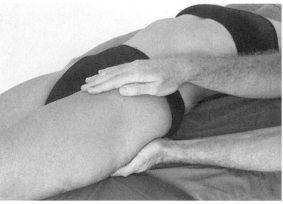

Figure 15.21. Hip bones supine c

The contact with the bottom hand is resting on the table. It is very important that the top hand be propped under the elbow with a pillow (just beyond the frame of Figures 15.20 and 15.21).

The practitioner's body is turned and looking diagonally toward the opposite leg and foot of the client.

Hip with Knees in Flexion

Window: The practitioner makes bilateral contact with both ischial tuberosities of the client, as shown in Figures 15.22, 15.23, and 14.24. The knees of the client need to be flexed.

The client's knees are flexed and together. The client needs to have the feet splayed out laterally in order to have the knees rest together. Sometimes if the practitioner has long enough arms, the client's legs can be cradled together with the practitioner using her shoulder and opposite arm for cradling the client's legs.

Summary: This is a wonderful way to help a pregnant woman increase the flexibility of her pelvis in preparation for birth. The practitioner is sensing the midline of the client's pelvis either through the vagina of a woman or the penis of a man breathing with Primary Respiration. This skill helps clarify the pelvic midline, especially for a woman who is pregnant (the baby becomes familiar with his or her escape route). For a man this can help the prostate breathe with Primary Respiration. As an alternative, the client can sit on the edge of

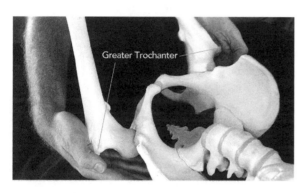

Figure 15.22. Hip in flexion a

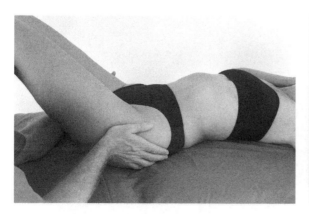

Figure 15.23. Hip in flexion b

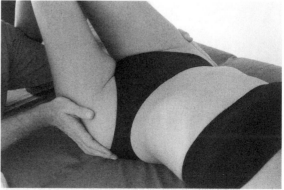

Figure 15.24. Hip in flexion c

the table and the practitioner can make bilateral contact with the client's ischial tuberosities from behind the client.

Coccyx

Window: The practitioner places the pad of one finger in proximity to the client's coccyx, similar to Figure 15.7 and Figure 15.8. Except here, the practitioner's free hand rests in her lap.

She senses any one of the following possibilities: PR, intraosseous sacral movement in PR, the longitudinal fluctuation of the fluid body, or the inherent motion of the neural tube.

This is where the primitive streak begins at the third week postfertilization. The longitudinal fluctuation of the fluid body is what initiates the primitive streak.

This position is also specific to the notochordal midline of the body and therefore essential to biodynamic practice. The midline here refers to the fluid midline of the longitudinal fluctuation and the notochord that results from the primitive streak activity. This is crucial for decompressing the central nervous system.

Longitudinal Fluctuation

It is highly recommended to have a thorough intake on the client, including any history of physical or sexual abuse. Health-related issues concerning the intestines and pelvic organs should be known as well as prescribed medications currently being taken. These preexisting conditions dampen or greatly reduce the longitudinal fluctuation (LF). The LF is the midline of the fluid body and therefore crucial to its rehabilitation. Traditionally the LF is considered to be associated with the ascent of the cerebrospinal fluid starting at the coccyx going through the core link (dura mater) and ending in the third ventricle. The descent of the fluctuating cerebrospinal fluid starts at the ethmoid bone and recedes back to the coccyx. This can be sensed when using the core link window.

Because of the high concentration of organic magnetic material in the dura mater, the cerebrospinal fluid is considered to have a bioelectric magnetic field associated with it. Numerous practitioners have experienced a second avenue of descent in the LF that goes out of the head much like a fountain and then cascades down and around the skin in an envelope 15–20 inches off the skin and finally reforming at the coccyx. Perhaps this is why Dr. Sutherland called it the "direct current." The rate of the LF is very precise at two and a half cycles per minute (2.5 CPM).

Process: The client is supine and the practitioner is sitting at the client's side at an angle, facing the client's head and neck.

The practitioner settles into an awareness of her own pelvic floor and may even initiate a few Kegel exercises in herself. A Kegel is a slight tightening of the muscles of the pelvic floor as if holding back from urinating or defecating. Alternatively, the practitioner can breathe down between the umbilicus and pubic bone in order to soften the pelvic floor and create space between the pubic bone and coccyx from anterior to posterior and the two ischial tuberosities from lateral to medial. Either way, the intention is to initiate an awareness of the LF in the practitioner first.

Practitioner synchronizes her secondary and PR and waits for zone C or D to become still.

Practitioner may sense the receding of the LF in the middle of her fluid body.

Alternatively, the practitioner visualizes her own LF from the coccyx to the third ventricle and the return in zone B as a fountain that then reforms at the coccyx.

Practitioner negotiates permission to make contact with her index or middle finger of the hand closest to the client and makes contact with the space around the coccyx and S5, as shown in Figures 15.7 and 15.8. The finger touches the bone in that area. The other hand may contact the client's sacral base (but that may be too much depending on the client's history).

The practitioner reorients, resynchronizes, and reattunes to her fluid body and the horizon.

The practitioner synchronizes attention with the health and wholeness (Primary Respiration) of the client's fluid body.

The practitioner may ask the client to visualize the anatomical space in his body from the coccyx up through the spine all the way to the middle of the brain. Rather than ask the client to sense his zone B, ask the client to sense his skin and then either the outside surface of the skin or the inside surface. Each step of the way, the practitioner must remember that there are two possibilities for the return and both are equal in therapeutic value.

The practitioner waits to sense the 2.5 CPM movement of the LF in the client. It moves twelve seconds from the coccyx to the third ventricle, returns for twelve seconds as it goes straight back down from the ethmoid or out around zone B, and starts the cycle again up from the coccyx. During the return, the practitioner waits in zone B or her own fluid body core sensing the ebb and flow of her LF.

Upon sensing the LF, the practitioner moves her attention to the central stillness within the LF. Wait for the potency and permeation of the LF to clarify and or ignite its therapeutic intention three dimensionally.

Gradually, the practitioner moves her attention out to the horizon and synchronizes with the interchange between stillness and Primary Respiration.

An alternative way to complete the exploration of the LF is to switch the client into sidelying and sense the LF via the notochord window, discussed in the next chapter.

Summary: The presence of the LF is an important evaluation in the sense that it is frequently missing in the contemporary client due to traumatic stress, lifestyle, surgery, medication, and chronic inflammatory conditions (see Chapters 1 through 4). Just as the fluid body has a pulse associated with Primary Respiration, so too the LF is the midline pulse of the fluid body with a faster tempo. Its pulse also needs to be checked early in a session and then again at the end of a session, just as an acupuncturist checks a client's meridian pulses at the beginning and end of a session. When the LF pulse is weak or unavailable, the focus is upon the pulse of the whole three-dimensional fluid body and its ability to breathe and be augmented with Primary Respiration. Then the practitioner waits for the LF to ignite by periodically returning to it in subsequent sessions by establishing a resonance in the practitioner's body, as described above.

The pulse of the fourth ventricle via the traditional CV4 window may need to be taken around the occipitomastoid suture, which Dr. Becker claimed as the premier gateway to the fourth ventricle. The pulse of the third ventricle may also need to evaluated. Both of these pulses are discussed in Chapter 18. The lateral fluctuation of the fluids in the cranium is in direct relationship with the LF. Consequently, the lateral fluctuations are an important pulse. When the lateral fluctuation in the cranium is very strong it may indicate a weakness in the LF, which means that the lateral fluctuation is overcompensating. The restoration of a balanced LF and lateral fluctuation very much depends on the overall balance of these fluid body pulses just mentioned. Practically, I would invite the clinician to become familiar with the EV4 as I outline in both Chapters 16 and 18. The EV4 is an excellent way to begin rebalancing the LF and lateral fluctuations.

Although it may seem unconventional, numerous sex therapists recommend masturbation to orgasm for both men and women as a way to reinhabit or revitalize the pelvis and thus the LF from a biodynamic point of view. An inability to orgasm (preorgasmic), painful intercourse, and generalized pain in the pelvis may not only be related to early childhood abuse but directly related to the extinguishing of the LF. Such exploration must be done with a qualified sex therapist or psychotherapist. It is unethical for a manual therapist to explore such issues with a client.

I will also recommend a series of colonic irrigation treatments for anyone who is chronically constipated. Constipation reduces the potency of the LF and the orgasm reflex in general. Gut and pelvic floor issues are epidemic in the culture and greatly reduce the functioning of the fluid body. Many pelvic issues cannot be cured by manual therapy alone but can be greatly helped with a sensitive and well-bounded practitioner. All work around the pelvis must be done with this understanding and a great sensibility while maintaining awareness of the whole with Primary Respiration.

CHAPTER 16

The Spine, Trunk, and Neck

The Snake

Window: The client is supine. The practitioner sits at the side of the client and places his hands under the thoracic spine between the scapulae or below them depending on the size of one's hands (see Figures 16.1 and 16.2). Both hands are palm up around the mid to lower thoracic spine of the client with the spinous processes of the client's vertebra in the fingers or in the palm of the practitioner, depending on the client's comfort.

Process: The practitioner comes into relationship with thoracic respiration in himself and then the client. He then drops his attention to the stillness and/or motion of the client's notochord, either two dimensionally on the long axis or three dimensionally.

The practitioner senses the serpentine movement of the notochord or the stillness of the notochord. Stillness is the deepest part of the embryonic core. The embryo orients its growth to the stillness, which is in the middle of the cellular structure of the notochord and throughout the body in various tissue

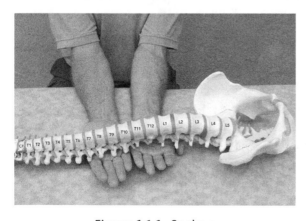

Figure 16.1. Snake a

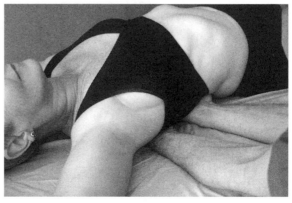

Figure 16.2. Snake b

and vascular structures. There is a natural biological quietness throughout the human body essential to growth and development.

Summary: This process begins to normalize the ANS, breathing, and cardiovascular functions in the client. It is especially good for clients who spend a lot of time hunched over a computer.

Primordial Breath

Window: Practitioner's hands are together under the crura of the respiratory diaphragm, palm up, with one hand above T12 and one hand below. This part of the diaphragm starts inside the body wall in the embryo along with the floating ribs. It is important to take into consideration the floating ribs in the hand that is located superiorly. Figure 16.1 also illustrates the proximity of the hands, which are similar in placement as with the Snake.

Process: The practitioner senses the diaphragmatic breathing of the client in three phases:

- Beginning with the actual structures of the tissue and bones, the practitioner gets a sense of the motion present in the musculoskeletal system in that area.

- Then the practitioner moves deeper into sensing the physiology of the ANS within the diaphragm. How do the brain, heart, and lungs work together in relation to nerve impulses coming from the brain and heart and also the gut?

- Then the practitioner moves his attention to the whole three-dimensional fluid body of the client and lets go of the previous two sensibilities. The practitioner senses the primordial origin of the breathing function through an image. Is it a water creature or a land animal? The practitioner waits until an image arises in his mind's eye and then is finished.

Meanwhile, the practitioner is synchronizing Primary Respiration (PR) with his secondary respiration. It directly relates to the ignition process. It is vital that Primary and secondary respiration be synchronized.

Summary: This practice induces a deep stillness and opens the heart. It begins to allow the client to breathe with the natural world. By sensing the ancient function of breathing, the fluid body is able to reconnect with its origin, which is essential for a client to renew herself.

Lungs

Window: Figure 16.3 shows my hands bilaterally on the costal arch of the ribs. This is the way I like to sense Primary Respiration moving the lungs. Primary Respiration breathes the lungs toward its original point between the third and fifth cervical vertebra. This is where the lungs originated in the embryo. From the vantage point of the costal arch, I can sense Primary Respiration breathing the lungs back and forth from the lower cervical spine. I like to either stand for this hand position or sit on the edge of the treatment table.

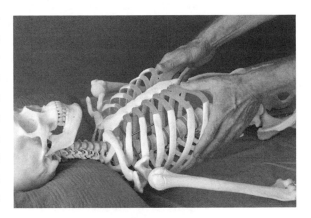

Figure 16.3. Lungs

The Notochord

Window: The client is in a sidelying position, her head supported with a pillow. It does not matter whether the client is lying on her right or left side. It could be important to offer the client a choice as to which side she prefers to lie on.

The other important postural component of this exploration is that the practitioner's arms and shoulders will be slightly lower or slightly beneath the plane of the top of the treatment table. When I practice this in my office, I frequently sit on a meditation cushion on the floor so that my hands can easily contact the top and bottom of the notochord without any strain in the wrist. This will take some time to set up the right position for each individual practitioner, because the critical component is strain in the wrist and shoulder-neck tension in the practitioner. This must be avoided.

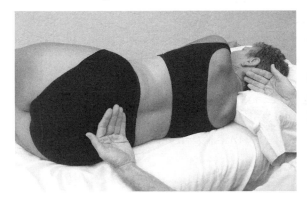

Figure 16.4. Notochord a

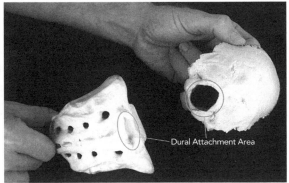

Figure 16.5. Notochord b

Process: The practitioner establishes the intersubjective field of orienting, synchronizing, and attuning. Relating with the notochord requires the practitioner to refine his skills of apprehending the inside presence of PR in his own fluid body as well as that of the client. To do this, the simplest area of concentration is on the spine. Once the practitioner has established a sense and shape or image of three-dimensional buoyancy in his own fluid body, then he brings subtle attention to the entire length of his spine from the coccyx up through the basiocciput and basisphenoid. In the osteopathic tradition, the basiocciput and basisphenoid are considered to be the top two vertebra of the spine and indeed are formed from the tip of the notochord embryologically.

PR has several two-dimensional vectors that it moves on and around the spine. The first vector sensed in the notochord of the spine comes from the top of the head straight down the spine for fifty seconds and then changes direction, coming right up from the earth through the pelvis and right through the top of the head for fifty seconds.

A second vector is one that I tend to focus on, the embryonic vector. This vector is like an accordion opening and closing for fifty seconds each way. The top of the accordion is actually the basisphenoid around the front of the face and the bottom of the accordion is the coccyx. When the accordion opens it causes a very slight sense of the spine lengthening and flexing. The head will also feel like it is slightly bowing with micro movement. Then when PR reverses itself and the notochordal midline shortens, there will be a slight sensation of the spine and head going into extension.

The structure in osteopathy called the core link is relevant to working with the notochord. The core link relates to the dural attachment around the foramen magnum of the occiput and second sacral segment, as shown in Figure 16.5. The core link, the notochord, the longitudinal fluctuation, the movement of cerebrospinal fluid, and the movement of the neural tissue itself are all valid entry points for exploring the structural midline of the client. A practitioner over time gathers the necessary experience to distinguish these various levels of motion (see Appendix) present in the client. The breathing of Primary Respiration in the notochord will not always be available to the practitioner.

That being said, the practitioner should always be ready to allow PR to teach him something he does not know. It is always willing to show the humble practitioner another dimension of its therapeutic activity of generating, repairing, and maintaining the human body.

Once the practitioner is comfortable with the inside presence of PR in his own fluid body, he requests permission to make contact with the client's occiput and sacrum.

I typically will use the back of my hands on the client's occiput and sacrum, as shown in Figure 16.4, rather than the palms of my hands. When I use the palms of my hands, it tends to bend my wrists and creates strain within seconds.

Now the practice is the same in the sense of becoming receptive and reorienting, resynchronizing, and reattuning with the interpersonal space and beyond to the natural world and back. The practitioner waits for PR to reveal which vector in the client's notochordal midline it wants to show, then attends to several cycles of Primary Respiration.

There are no photographs for this step. Once the practitioner has noticed several cycles, he will switch the hand on the occiput to a very light, single-finger contact over the glabella of the client. From this vantage point the practitioner may be able to sense the receding of the longitudinal fluctuation going back down to the coccyx.

Once the practitioner creates a bigger wing span with his arms, he will need to sit higher up than when in contact with the sacrum and occiput. Now he will need to sit in a regular chair or stool.

The glabella is the center of the forehead between the eyebrows and slightly above the bridge of the nose. Once again, he is on the very top of the notochordal midline because the sphenoid is posterior to the finger on the glabella.

The bottom hand on the sacrum switches down closer to the coccyx. In this way, the practitioner's hands span the entire length of the adult remnants of the notochordal midline. At this point, the process is the same as above. Reorient, resynchronize, and reattune until PR reveals itself once again.

It is important to solicit the comfort of the client because of the finger position on the face. The practitioner makes sure that his arms and wrists are well supported by the table or other pillows.

Summary: This is actually a great way to end the session with the client. It is not only very relaxing, but decompresses the autonomic nervous system and offers some insurance if there were any side effects from the session the client just received. It is not enough to be able to sense PR. The practitioner must also be able to establish a conscious relationship with the interchange that PR has with Dynamic Stillness that permeates the office space. It is the type of stillness that is filled with precision, clarity, and nonthought. This allows the fluid body to go into a neutral. The neutral is the way in which the fluid body pauses its motion and reestablishes its own relationship with a dynamic field of stillness that not only exists within it, but three dimensionally all around it.

Respiratory Diaphragm

Window: Practitioner is seated at the side of the table and places both hands together, palm up under the client's spine, with T12–L1 located at the junction of the right and left hand. Figures 16.1 and 16.2 illustrate this position.

The exploration is to begin to sense the relationship of PR to secondary respiration.

The diaphragm is a door, so to speak, to the heart and can modify the behavior of the heart through the respiratory sinus arrhythmia relationship between the diaphragm and heart, which developed prenatally.

The diaphragm is not only related to the heart and PR, but also is the fulcrum for the fluid body, according to some osteopaths. Secondary respiration is always a fundamental consideration in every biodynamic session.

The practitioner might occasionally direct the client to breathe between her umbilicus and pubic bone. This is only done a couple of times in any given session.

Shoulders (Heart Holding)

Window: The practitioner sits at the head of the table. Gently negotiate permission to make contact and place the hands buoyantly over the shoulders bilaterally, as shown in Figure 16.6.

Practitioner lets PR choose which shoulder to focus on.

The practitioner then sits at the side of the table and is still. The client is supine and the practitioner's body is perpendicular to the client's shoulder.

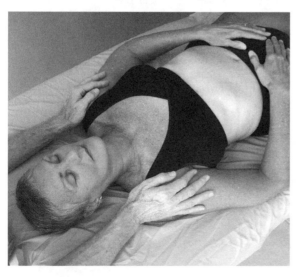

Figure 16.6. Bilateral shoulders

Process: The practitioner contemplates stillness in his body, in the office space, and out the window with the eyes open. Alternatively, the practitioner may focus on stillness in his body with eyes closed.

The practitioner connects with the earth by relaxing through the pelvis and feeling the heat of the earth 100 miles or more below while PR is breathing itself into the floor of the pelvis, filling the fluid body and returning back down into the earth every fifty seconds.

The practitioner senses the client with the heart mirror, especially if approaching the client's left shoulder where the heart is located.

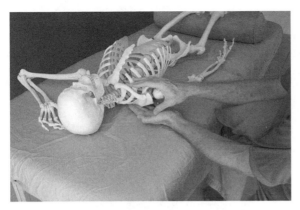

Figure 16.7. Ipsilateral shoulder a

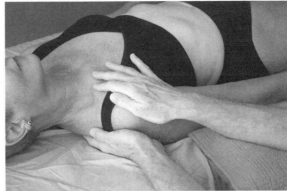

Figure 16.8. Ipsilateral shoulder b

The practitioner makes contact with one shoulder of the client ipsilaterally, as if holding a bowl of water. One hand is under the scapula and the other is floating over the clavicle and humeral head (see Figures 16.7 and 16.8).

Allow PR to breathe through each shoulder especially through the heart when in contact with the left shoulder. This will allow the heart muscles and related ligamentous structures to decompress from traumatic impact injuries to the region of the thorax or other related shocks, such as explosions that soldiers experience in war.

Summary: The timing of PR is not the most important aspect of its activity. It is just a convenient way for some practitioners to enter into its healing presence. It is more important to sense PR changing directions to observe ignition. This is a wonderful way to relate to those clients with shoulder issues. It is helpful for upper lung freedom and the upper three ribs as well. It is also a good way to approach the head and neck. Finally, when the practitioner is on the client's left shoulder she is also holding the heart of the client and can help the heart relax and open.

Clavicles

The clavicles form in the fetal period and are a distinct human structure related to a proper cervical and lumbar curve. The clavicles are the base of the pharyngeal arches and thus are the gateway to the face biodynamically.

The clavicles and their fascia directly relate to the thoracic duct of the lymphatic system, the vagus nerve, the subclavian vein and arteries, and the carotid arteries. This can be very soothing for the autonomic nervous system (ANS) and help lymphatic drainage from the head and neck.

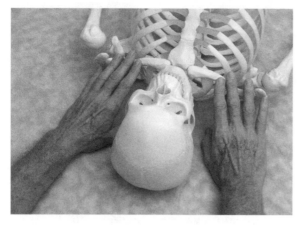

Figure 16.9. Clavicles a

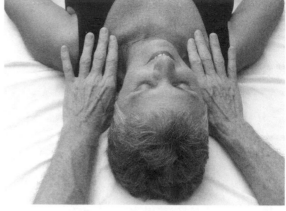

Figure 16.10. Clavicles b

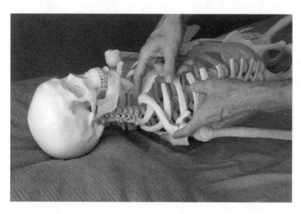

Figure 16.11. Clavicles c

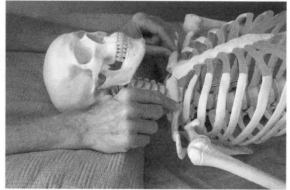

Figure 16.12. Clavicles d

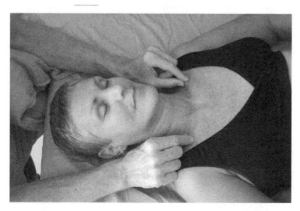

Figure 16.13. Clavicles e

Window: Practitioner is seated at the head of the table. Hands are palm down. The index, middle, and ring fingers are bilaterally spanning each clavicle, as shown in Figures 16.9 and 16.10. Only the finger pads make contact starting at midclavicle. The thumbs are resting gently around the head of first ribs and possibly the spine without any compression.

This bilateral hand configuration allows the practitioner to sense PR around the midline, as well as balanced bilateral movement of the clavicles and any intraosseous restrictions.

Gradually, the practitioner senses the lymphatic and vascular systems so close to his hands. The blood moves in spirals through canalization zones under the clavicles and medial to the sternocleidomastoid muscles in the neck. In addition the heart was originally located in the neck and grew down into its adult placement by the end of the embryonic period. The practitioner listens to the blood and early heart located in the neck as it passes through the thoracic inlet under the clavicles.

It helps to imagine that the client's neck is like a tubular sea sponge that simply gets wider at the clavicles. In this way everything experienced inside the sea sponge can occur in the tempo of Primary Respiration.

Figure 16.11 shows my index fingers contacting the distal and proximal heads of the right clavicle. If the client has one clavicle that is more symptomatic than the other, then explore the one side as shown with Primary Respiration as it breathes between the fingers.

Following the exploration of one clavicle the practitioner reorients to both clavicles. The contact is made with the tissue-plucking hand position shown in Figures 16.12 and 16.13. The index fingers and thumbs are together and the tips of the fingers are making bilateral contact with the middle of the client's clavicles. Here the various motions of the clavicles become more readily available with PR and both clavicles have the opportunity to come into balance.

The general skill is to sense layers of the body from the outer osseous to the inner vascular component and then back out to the clavicles being breathed by Primary Respiration.

Pleura

This hand position is for contacting the cervical pleural ligament as it attaches on the pleura of the lungs. It is also the originating point of the lungs in the embryo. In the adult, the pleura is suspended from the cervical spine as high up as the third cervical vertebra in the neck.

Window: Here my fingers are located by the transverse processes of the mid to lower cervical spine, as shown in Figure 16.14. I like to wait and just sense all the tissues melting with PR. Gradually, the client's breathing will expand the upper lobes of the lungs and consequently the pleura, which can be readily sensed with the fingers.

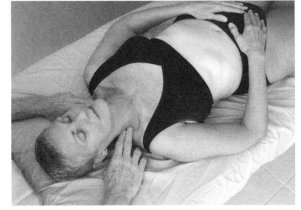

This is the embryonic fulcrum for the lungs and a very important window to view the activity of PR in the core of the body.

Figure 16.14. Pleura

Heart Fulcrum

This exploration is to sense the embryonic fulcrum of the heart and balance the space above and below the foramen magnum. The heart starts in the neck region of the embryo around the third and fourth cervical vertebrae (C3–C4). This is the original fulcrum of the embryonic heart. The heart then grows down into the trunk as development unfolds.

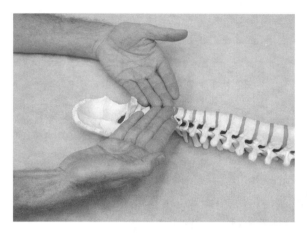

Figure 16.15. Heart fulcrum a

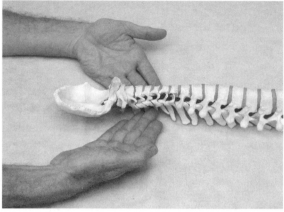

Figure 16.16. Heart fulcrum b

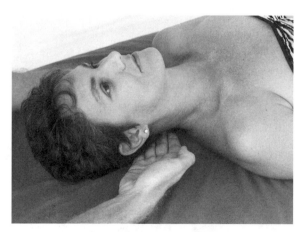

Figure 16.17. Heart fulcrum c

Window: The client is supine. Practitioner is seated above the head of the client and places the index and or middle fingertips together under the nape of the neck around the third and fourth cervical vertebrae (C3–C4). The hands are palm up, as shown in Figures 16.15, 16.16, and 16.17. Note that the practitioner's fingertips are touching when actually under the neck. Figure 16.15 is showing that togetherness above the neck, for visibility.

The practitioner orients to PR breathing through the heart fulcrum from posterior to anterior. In other words, the breathing proceeds from the table up to the ceiling and back rather than longitudinally up and down the midline of the spine.

Summary: This balances the head with the rest of the body via the cardiovascular system when sensing PR moving posterior to anterior through this fulcrum. This window usually precedes any exploration on the head itself. It is very calming for the client.

Scapular EV4

This exploration is to sense the heart and thus the parasympathetic nervous system breathing with PR and/or a Mid Tide tempo. The Mid Tide tempo I usually sense is about one cycle per minute (CPM).

The scapulae are the hard coverings of the back of the heart; they help connect the hands and arms with the heart.

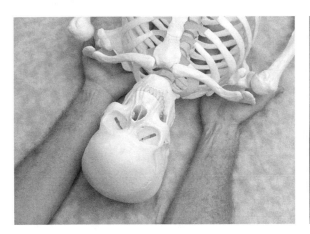

Figure 16.18. Scapular EV4 a

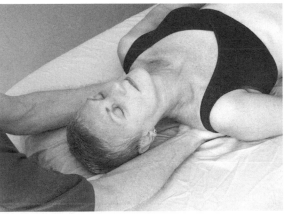

Figure 16.19. Scapular EV4 b

Window: The client is supine. Practitioner is seated above the head of the client and places one of the client's scapulae in each hand, as shown in Figures 16.18, 16.19, and 16.20. The practitioner must remember to turn his head and not breathe onto the client's face.

Summary: Frequently, the practitioner will perceive the rate of thirty seconds of expansion and thirty seconds of contraction (1 CPM) at the scapulae. Some osteopaths have called this rate the *reciprocal tension potency* of the fluid body. When synchronized with that rate there will be a tendency in the client's fluid body to

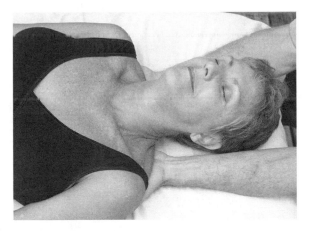

Figure 16.20. Scapular EV4 c

stillpoint at the end point of its expansion phase and thus the term EV4, which indicates such a stillpoint at the end of an expansion phase. There are some cases in which a stillpoint occurs at the end point of the contraction phase but that is much less frequent in the contemporary client because there is so much imprinted trauma in the client's midline. Consequently, a stillpoint in the expansion phase is much more gentle and permeates the fluid body systemically. This stillpoint will then shift into the fluid body systemically breathing with PR. This is very beneficial for the entire ANS.

Arms and Hands

Fear in the body is regulated through a brain structure called the amygdala. This hand position helps the amygdala to reduce its fear. It helps to balance the ANS and normalize traumatic stress.

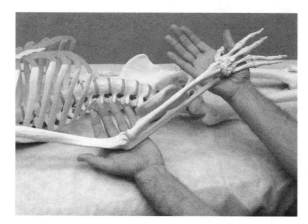

Figure 16.21. Arms and hands a

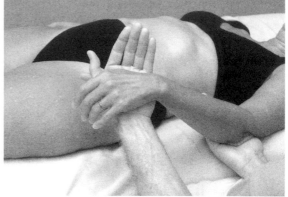

Figure 16.22. Arms and hands b

Window: Client can be seated or supine or even standing. The client's hand is placed palm down in the palm of the practitioner's hand. The free hand of the practitioner is placed under the elbow, as shown in Figures 16.21 and 16.22.

When the practitioner senses PR he moves the hand from under the elbow up to the shoulder or in back of the client's heart on the spine around T5, as shown in Figures 16.23 and 16.24. Synchronize attention again with PR.

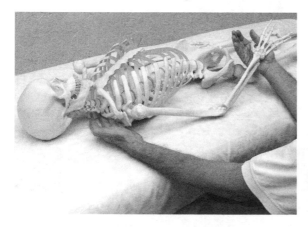

Figure 16.23. Arms and hands c

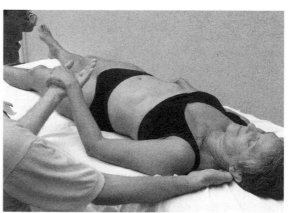

Figure 16.24. Arms and hands d

Repeat on the other hand, arm, and shoulder of the client.

Process: The client's comfort must be solicited periodically while performing this exploration. If the client expresses any discomfort, the practitioner asks the client to grip his hand more firmly and slightly push her arm into the practitioner's hand. The practitioner offers a little resistance for fifteen to thirty seconds and then releases the arm and hand of the client and waits for the client's ANS to settle. If this does not help, this exploration must be finished.

Atlas-Occiput Space

One of the nicest effects of these atlas-occiput space (AOS) explorations is the settling of the entire autonomic nervous system. This is the principal reason I use them in clinical practice.

The point of contact is the tip of the middle fingers (or others that are a better fit for the individual) of the practitioner in the AOS between the occiput and the second cervical vertebra. In this position, the practitioner's fingers are in contact with the superior cervical sympathetic ganglion. In addition, the fascia and muscle fibers of the suboccipital triangle actually go through the occiput and insert on the dura mater that covers the brain. This fascia is located just above the foramen magnum, as shown in Figure 16.25. Thus, the AOS palpation skills are exceedingly important.

The client is supine in the exploration variations described below, with the practitioner seated at the head of the client. The client's knees are flexed and resting together without any tension. If for some reason, the client's AOS is not responsive then try having the client's legs straight out with a pillow under the knees.

Variation 1

The first step is to get the practitioner's hands together into a proper position, as shown in Figure 16.26. The practitioner's initial exploration is to slide his hands under the top of the client's neck with the pads of the pinky and ring fingers contacting the space of the suboccipital triangle of muscles and squama of the occiput. The rest of the finger pads are in the nape of the neck. The practitioner senses that whole area before getting more specific.

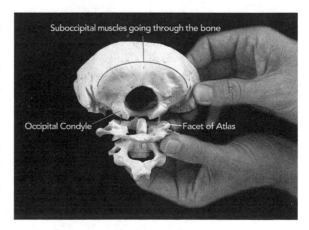

Figure 16.25. Atlas-occiput a

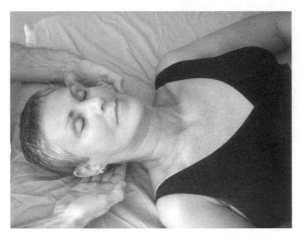

Figure 16.26. Atlas-occiput b

One important palpation skill for the AOS is to notice if there is any lymph edema there. It has a sense of the tissue being thick and spongy as if filled with too much fluid. This is usually the result of congestion from a whiplash injury or other types of neck or head injuries. Dr. Sutherland was in the habit of always making sure the lymphatic ducts were open in the neck and thoracic outlet area when he worked with the cranium. The practitioner must help drain the lymph before proceeding or refer the client for lymph drainage if there is such congestion in the AOS.

Variation 2

The practitioner lifts the client's head gently and rests it comfortably in his hands. The practitioner's ring and little fingers slightly overlap in such a way that the edges of the middle fingers (or, depending on the size of the practitioner's hands, the index fingers) come together. Figures 16.27, 16.28, and 16.29 show the precise finger positioning.

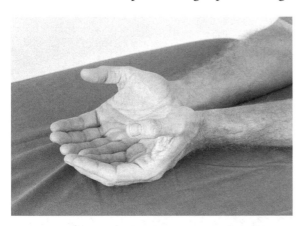

Figure 16.27. Atlas-occiput c

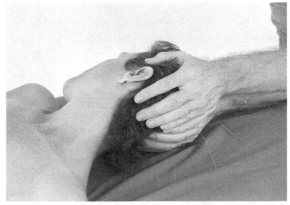

Figure 16.28. Atlas-occiput d

When placing the hands in this way under the client's head, the whole cranium of the client is cradled more or less in the medial aspects of the palms of the practitioner's hands. The *tips* of the middle fingers are used to discover the space between the occiput and the second cervical vertebra, C2. This is the center of the AOS. The atlas (C1) has no spinous process and consequently there is a gap between the occiput and C2. The *pads* of the middle fingers of the practitioner are resting against the client's occiput.

The practitioner softly cradles the client's head with full contoured contact of the client's cranium in the palms and hands of the practitioner.

After the practitioner reorients and resynchronizes, he slightly and gently curls the tips of the middle fingers back, as shown in Figures 16.30 and 16.31. This moves the client's chin ever so slightly into extension. If the client's neck is too stiff, the chin and cranium will not go into a slight extension. This is no problem and the

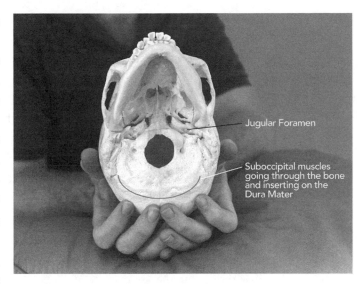

Figure 16.29. Atlas-occiput e

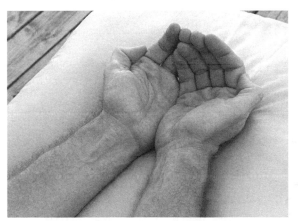

Figure 16.30. Atlas-occiput f

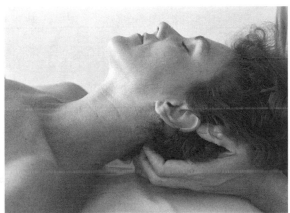

Figure 16.31. Atlas-occiput g

practitioner must not attempt to force or push the client's head into extension. In such a case I would recommend that the client have some soft-tissue work done on her neck before the next cranial session.

Next, the tips of the middle fingers begin to wedge slightly into the AOS with more firmness. Again, the practitioner needs to listen locally and globally for a minute or so during each stage of this process. This is because the muscles of the suboccipital triangle will soften gradually and usually soften one side at a time and the fluid body and ANS need time to get in register with the other layers. Consequently, the practitioner must keep accommodating to the motion of the client's head when the soft tissue relaxes on both sides. In other words, as the tissue softens the practitioner *takes up the slack* in the tissues by allowing his fingertips to move up into the AOS without excessive pressure but staying at the edge of any barriers encountered.

Variation 3

While cradling the AOS with the tips of the middle fingers, a figure eight may be explored through the fluid body of the practitioner into the suboccipital triangle of the client in the tempo of Primary Respiration. In other words, the practitioner begins to move his whole fluid body very subtly like a snake writhing or dancing in a figure eight. That motion translates through the hands of the practitioner into the AOS of the client. The practitioner periodically stops his motion and listens locally and out to the horizon. The basic motion in the fluid body is a spiral and the figure eight helps to amplify the therapeutic properties of the spiral.

The motions of the figure eight and tractioning are done with the whole hands and fluid body of the practitioner, not just the fingertips.

- Motion test with a figure eight: slightly rotate head to right not more than a one-quarter inch.
- Sidebend head to direction of ease, with micro motion.
- Repeat sequences every two minutes while waiting between sequences. Maximum is three sequences.
- Wait and sense opening and lengthening through soft tissue.

Variation 4

Gently spread the middle fingers laterally by moving the elbows together. This influences the jugular foramen and relieves pressure on the vagus nerve and jugular vein.

Variation 5

This AOS exploration involves the orienting reflex and the head-righting reflex. All of the AOS explorations have the ability to recalibrate visual and auditory attention to an external stimuli. This is a reflex located in the proprioceptors of the upper cervical spine and the cranial nerve nuclei including the fifth cranial nerve. The *head-righting reflex* is associated with being able to rest one's visual gaze on the horizon. This same reflex is also related to the ability to turn the head and orient to novel stimuli in the environment, which is the *orienting reflex.* Both of these reflexes are compromised with traumatic stress and the head becomes separate from the body in terms of perception.

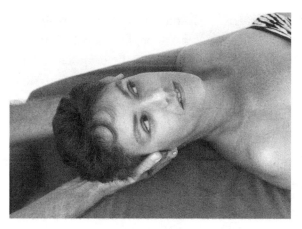

Figure 16.32. Atlas-occiput h

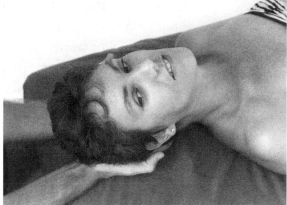

Figure 16.33. Atlas-occiput i

The practitioner asks the client to rotate her head to the left slowly and only a short distance (a couple of inches). Then the practitioner brings the client's head back to center and asks the client to turn her head to the right.

Now ask the client to look to the left and turn the head to the left, as shown in Figure 16.32.

Repeat the sequence, with the client looking this time to the right and turning the head to the right, as shown in Figure 16.33.

Bring the client's head to the center. This sequence can start with either direction, right or left.

Now the practitioner asks the client to look right while the practitioner rotates the client's head to the left. Note restrictions or motion barriers and stop when meeting a barrier and wait for it to soften.

Repeat the sequence to the opposite side.

This is a very powerful way to work. It should be attempted only after several sessions and only if the preceding variations are ineffective.

Variation 6

Place a microgram of traction on the occiput to explore the dura mater and any tension patterns it might be holding, especially from whiplash injuries. This is a very delicate traction that is done for several seconds and then released. Figure 16.34 shows the position of the fingers on the occiput.

This variation is a visualization exploration. The practitioner visualizes the dura mater and

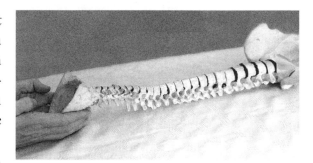

Figure 16.34. Atlas-occiput-dural tube traction

subarachnoid space that is filled with cerebrospinal fluid on the inside and attached to the vertebrae on the outside via the denticulate ligaments starting at the foramen magnum. Repeat several times or until the practitioner senses he is at the sacral attachment of the dura mater. It is barely an intention to traction. The tractional force is measured in nanograms!

It is also helpful to visualize the dural tube with its denticulate ligaments and subarachnoid space full of cerebrospinal fluid. In addition, the blood vascular supply to the meninges can be visualized as if the dura was pink and red.

- Offer a nanogram of traction for fifteen to thirty seconds on the occiput.

- Slowly count down the vertebrae from the first cervical all the way to the second sacral segment.

- Relax intention and wait fifteen to thirty seconds when noticing a tension or restriction in the dura mater. Practice moving attention out through the zones and back.

- Let the dura mater soften before moving on or simply go around the restriction if it chooses to remain.

- Repeat until sensing the dural tube attachment at the sacrum. In some clients I have continued down to the feet to imagine the client's body becoming like seaweed.

- Finally, fill the subarachnoid space and dura mater with a beautiful pink light from the cardiovascular system.

Caution must always be used with visualizations involving the inside of a client's body. The practitioner must be able to sense if the client is reacting to the visualization usually through a tissue contraction or the fluid body becoming tense. If softening and lengthening of the dura mater do not start occurring with a minute or two, the practitioner must abandon the visualization.

Process: One of the common mistakes is for the practitioner to relax the fingertips, whereas it is important to *take up the slack* as the suboccipital triangle softens as I mentioned. In this way, the atlas can begin to reseat itself onto the occipital condyles and a proper relationship along the whole suture line between the occiput and temporal bone can occur. Also, it is taught in the French osteopathic schools that the client's knees must be flexed for work in and around the AOS. I recommend trying both ways, with knees flexed and without, and see which is better for that client. Frequently my clients go fast asleep when my fingers are engaged in the AOS and consequently the knees must be well supported and without held tension in the legs if they are flexed.

I find that, when a client is highly toned sympathetically, if I start with an AOS exploration, it makes it much easier to sense the fluid body and tidal body. This is a judgment call on the part of the practitioner that requires skill and practice.

The biodynamic practitioner starts with the whole and in the middle of a session may move to more functional explorations if invited to do so. Nonetheless, every session begins and ends biodynamically. In other words, the best time to explore the AOS is in the middle of a session.

Summary: Contact is made with the superior cervical sympathetic ganglion in all the AOS variations. Trauma to the orienting reflex nerves may cause a person to have difficulty sensing her environment, which feels like an inability to easily turn the head or to rest attention on the horizon all the way to claustrophobic thinking and emotional breakdowns. This greatly interferes with the ability to perceive Primary Respiration from the horizon and back. It decreases one's ability to relate accurately with the environment, which is a hallmark of traumatic stress.

Finally, the occiput is the primary stress bone during a vaginal delivery. Three typical intraosseous patterns are imprinted in the occiput from birth: shelving, telescoping, and torsion. During exploration with the AOS, as well as the transverse sinus (covered in Chapter 17), it is possible to encounter these birth dynamics and normalize any intraosseous or interosseous stress imprinting from birth as long as the practitioner is synchronized with Primary Respiration.

Summary of AOS Variations

Variation 1:

- The practitioner gets a sense of the whole area of the upper neck with his finger pads.

Variation 2:

- Hands are positioned for an occiput cradle with middle fingers at AOS. Finger pads on occiput, tips of fingers toward body of atlas in soft tissue. Middle fingers are slightly curled back toward the atlas in the soft tissue area.

- Practitioner holds the head of the client like like a bowl of water and senses Primary Respiration.

- Practitioner may move fingertips to extend the client's chin very slightly if there is ease of movement.

Variation 3:

• Slowly move the whole head in a figure eight with micro movement.

Variation 4:

• The practitioner gently brings his elbows closer together to exert a lateral spreading of the fingers. This influences the client's jugular foramen to open and soften.

Variation 5:

• Client rotates head to one side, and then the other, slowly and only a couple of inches.

• Client moves eyes to right; practitioner turns head right several inches and back to midline. Repeat sequence, with client's eyes to left and moving head to left.

• Then have client look with her eyes to one side while rotating the head to the opposite side. Repeat this sequence, in the opposite direction.

• Repeat a maximum of three times or until opening and lengthening are sensed in the AOS and cervical spine down to the sacrum.

Variation 6:

• Visualize the dura mater and subarachnoid space.

• Offer a tiny bit of traction for fifteen to thirty seconds on the occiput.

• Slowly count down the vertebrae from the first cervical to the second sacral segment.

• Relax intention and wait fifteen to thirty seconds when noticing a tension or restriction in the dura mater. Practice moving attention out through the zones and back. Let the dura mater soften before moving on or simply go around the restriction if it remains.

• Repeat until sensing the dural tube attachment at the sacrum.

• Fill the subarachnoid space and dura mater with a beautiful pink light from the cardiovascular system.

Heart Tube

Window: Figures 16.35 and 16.36 show the practitioner making contact with the sternum on top and the upper thoracic spine below. The intention is to be able to sense the heart tube of the embryo expand three dimensionally and breathe with Primary Respiration. The heart tube is inside two envelopes of fascia. The outer layer or bag that holds the lungs and heart in place is called the mediastinum. Then the heart is suspended internally by its support fascia called the pericardium that was present in the embryo. The pericardium has suspensory ligaments to the sternum and ribs that are frequently tight from stress both physical and emotional.

The practitioner's body position is very important. The left elbow needs to be supported by a pillow. In addition, if the practitioner's head, which cannot be seen in the photos, is above or near the client's head, he will need to turn his head so that when he exhales, she does not feel the practitioner's breath on her face. This can be very distracting and uncomfortable for a client.

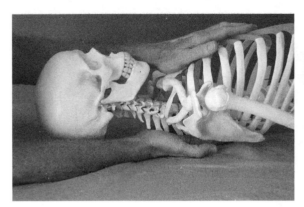

Figure 16.35. Heart tube a

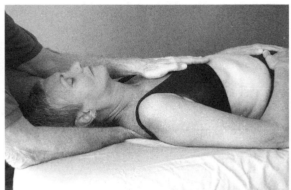

Figure 16.36. Heart tube b

Once the hands and arms are comfortable, the practitioner senses the movement of the respiratory diaphragm and how breathing moves the ribs and lungs.

Gradually, the practitioner senses the movement of the heart and toggles his attention back and forth between his heart movement and that of the client and then periodically moves attention out through the zones.

The heart tube wants to expand. That is its basic embryonic nature and the practitioner waits to sense Primary Respiration in the client's heart. This is a window that can be revisited more than once in a series of sessions.

Side effects may include a dull ache around the attachments of the suspensory ligaments of the heart to the rib cage, a general feeling of tightness in the thorax, elevated heart rate, or emotional release. These effects are usually transient and the practitioner must maintain focus on his own heart and ask the client to breathe slowly into an area of tightness.

Chapter 17

The Face

Mandible Developmental Movements

The foregut consists of the bones, muscles, and other embryological derivatives of the face, pharynx, and esophagus. In order to explore the face, a good starting position is to hold the client's mandible and sense its anterior-posterior and inferior-superior movement. The hand position recommended here will allow you to feel the two possible developmental movements of both the adult and the child. When an infant is breastfeeding the mandible moves anterior-posterior. Once a child begins to eat solid food the mandible moves inferiorly-superiorly, which persists into adulthood. Because hand size in relation to the client's face size is the determining factor in this window, remember to gauge one's hand placement accordingly.

Window: The practitioner sits at the head of the table and, after orienting, places the thenar eminences of her thumbs bilaterally on or near the condyles of the client's mandible, as shown in Figure 17.1. The tops of the thumbs are on the angle of the mandible bilaterally. The wrists and arms must be supported properly on the table to be able to relax both hands once a comfortable hand location has been found.

Summary: Remember to access the fluid fields of the embryo whenever on or around the face with Primary Respiration (PR). The sense of the developmental movement occurs when the anterior-posterior movements of the

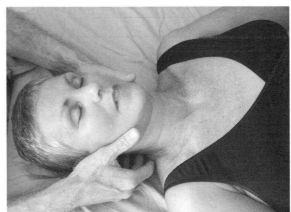

Figure 17.1. Mandible developmental movements

infant mandible balance with the inferior-superior movements of the adult mandible and typically a stillpoint is achieved. At this point, the bone itself may begin to breathe three dimensionally with PR. This exploration reflexes into the temporomandibular joint (TMJ) and the cranial base.

Face Seams

In these face windows, it must be remembered that throughout prenatal development and all the way through adolescence, the face is developing horizontally. Consequently, any palpation of the face is done with this sensitivity and quality of movement. Once young adulthood approaches, the face then moves into its vertical growth pattern. The face induces the heart and brain to grow as an embryo and consequently these seams are very important and usually precede exploration with the cranial base.

Practitioner has lateral contact on the client's face and neck. Practitioner's finger pads are in between the pharyngeal arch derivatives. The sequence is as follows:

- Hyoid bone (see Figures 17.2, 17.3, and 17.4)

- Mandible (see Figures 17.5, 17.6, and 17.7)

- Temporomandibular joint (TMJ) (see Figures 17.8 and 17.9)

- Maxilla (see Figures 17.10 and 17.11)

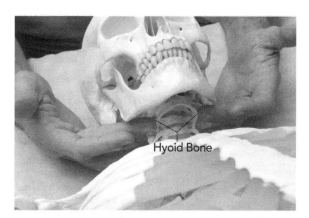

Figure 17.2. Hyoid bone a

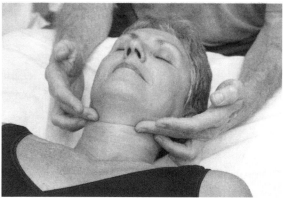

Figure 17.3. Hyoid bone b

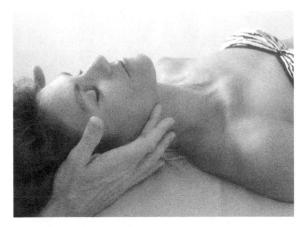

Figure 17.4. Hyoid bone c

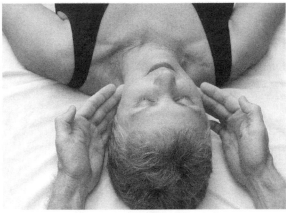

Figure 17.5. Mandible a

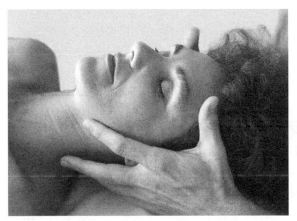

Figure 17.6. Mandible b

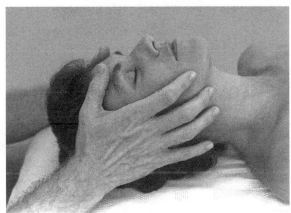

Figure 17.7. Mandible c

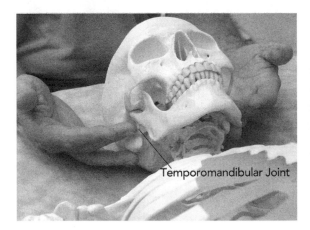

Temporomandibular Joint

Figure 17.8. Temporomandibular joint a

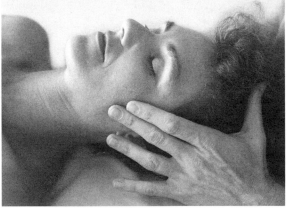

Figure 17.9. Temporomandibular joint b

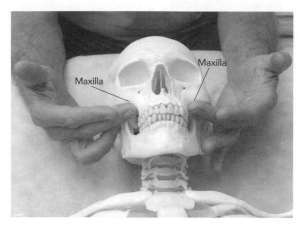

Figure 17.10. Maxilla a

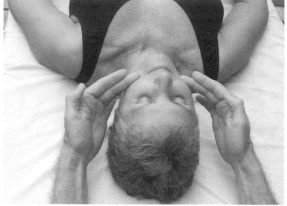

Figure 17.11. Maxilla b

Process:

1. Practitioner begins with her hands six inches lateral of the client's head in zone B and synchronizes her attention with PR in or around the client.

2. Practitioner verbally negotiates contact with the first seam starting at the hyoid and going sequentially from the bottom to the top of the face.

3. Practitioner orients to the stillness under her fingers.

4. Practitioner synchronizes with lateral-medial movements of the fluid body, or by its 3D breathing in PR.

5. Practitioner observes ignition phenomena if available. Care must be taken to ensure that the practitioner's hands and arms are well supported. The practitioner must remember to have her hands open and extended rather than flexed. The exploration is done with finger pads not fingertips.

Repeat steps 2, 3, and 4 with each seam.

Summary: As a way to complete the session, the practitioner may contact the fluid body with the Pietà position and wait for the whole fluid body to breathe with Primary Respiration. The sacrum is always a good option for ending any exploration around the head.

Transverse Sinus

Window: Figure 17.12 shows the practitioner's finger pads lined up to approximate the location of the client's transverse sinus. The transverse sinus is located on a line going from lateral to medial on the inner surface of the occiput. The external location of the finger pads is along that same line with the external occipital protuberance as the center point for the little or ring fingers depending on the size of the practitioner's hands.

The practitioner sits above the head of the client and senses softening in that area of the occiput while synchronized with PR.

The transverse sinus is formed by the superior and inferior leafs of the tentorium and consequently this is an excellent way to decompress the entire tentorium and assist the vascular system of the head to drain better.

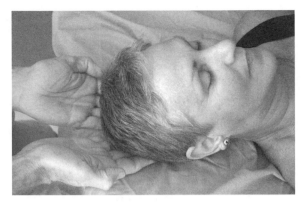

Figure 17.12. Transverse sinus

The Anterior-Posterior Fluid Fields of the Face

These windows are related to ignition in general and specifically the importance of the face in inducing the brain and heart embryonically.

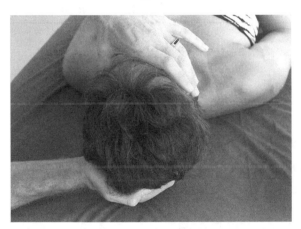

Figure 17.13. Anterior-posterior fluid fields a

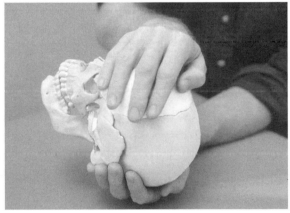

Figure 17.14. Anterior-posterior fluid fields b (photographed by Robert Cutter)

Window: Client is supine. Practitioner is sitting at the side perpendicular to the client's head.

The practitioner uses the hand opposite the top of the client's head and rests the client's occiput on the palm and/or fingers of her hand, as shown in Figures 17.13 and 17.14.

The client's external occipital protuberance is situated between the ring finger and middle finger of the practitioner. In this way, the middle finger of the practitioner approximates the superior leaf of the tentorium. The ring finger approximates the inferior leaf of the client's tentorium.

It is fine for the practitioner to use other fingers depending on the size of her hand.

Process: The intention is to wait until the practitioner can sense a spreading or gapping of the superior and inferior leaves of the tentorium.

Upon sensing the spreading of the tentorium, the practitioner makes contact with the client's upper fluid field with her free hand.

The practitioner's free hand is positioned in a way that the pad of the thumb and pad of the middle finger are in light contact with the lateral portion of the frontal bone of the client. The practitioner waits to sense PR breathing between her two hands.

Then the practitioner shifts her free hand to the maxillary fluid field in order to sense the same dynamic.

Then the practitioner switches her free hand to the mandibular fluid field.

Finally, the practitioner can use her free hand to sense the hyoid fluid field from front to back.

Summary: As an alternative, the practitioner can *stand* at the side of the client and use both hands to contact the hyoid-mandible fluid fields bilaterally, the mandibular maxillary fluid fields bilaterally, and finally the maxillary-frontal fluid fields bilaterally.

Ethmoid Bone

Window: There are many ways to make contact with the ethmoid bone. This window places the practitioner's thumb over the glabella of the frontal bone, as shown in Figure 17.15. The rest of the practitioner's hand is making a very light contact. As the fluid fields of the face breathe laterally, the thumbs will depress as if the hands were like wings. When PR changes direction, the reverse of that motion will occur. The ethmoid bone will lift the thumbs and the wings of the hands will settle down closer to the face.

Process: Many clients have had facial trauma and, occasionally, I mechanically attempt to loosen the ethmoid bone before balancing it biodynamically. The practitioner's left hand is cupping the client's frontal bone. The right hand is making contact with the lacrimal bones, as shown in Figure 17.16. The practitioner then induces a very gentle torsion motion. The left hand rotates one direction while the right hand goes in the opposite with perhaps several ounces of pressure. The practitioner will do this for several seconds in each direction, and then will stop and allow the face to breathe with PR.

Figure 17.17 shows the left hand in the same position cupping the frontal bone. The thumb and index finger of the right hand are making contact with the client's maxilla. The process is the same as in the previous paragraph. This hand position is done in conjunction with the previous one in order to get a more thorough sense of freedom in the ethmoid bone without using intraoral work.

Summary: It is important if using this type of skill to balance the fluid fields of the face with PR.

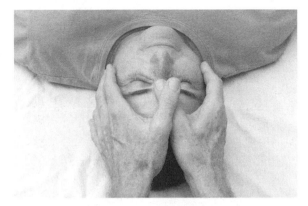

Figure 17.15. Ethmoid a (with Valerie Gora)

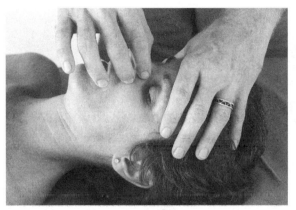

Figure 17.16. Ethmoid b

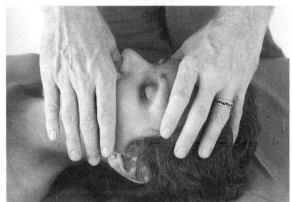

Figure 17.17. Ethmoid c

Intraorbital Ligament

The intraorbital ligament is responsible in prenatal development for pulling the eyes from the sides of the head into their normal anatomical position.

Window: This hand position combines a contact around the ethmoid with the pad of the left index finger and contact with the intraorbital ligament with the pad of the right index finger, as shown in Figure 17.18.

Figure 17.19 shows the practitioner's finger pads around the same position on the client's face. When synchronizing with PR at this level,

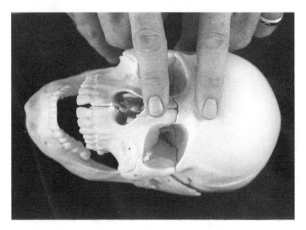

Figure 17.18. Intraorbital ligament a (photographed by Robert Cutter)

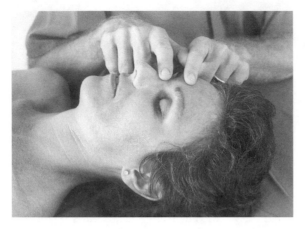

Figure 17.19. Intraorbital ligament b

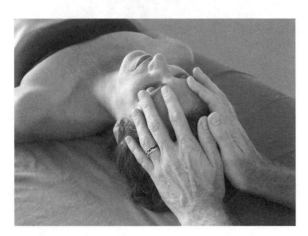

Figure 17.20. Frontal bone

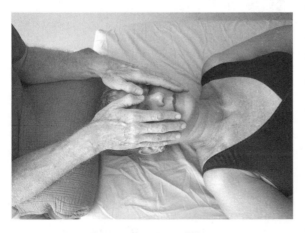

Figure 17.21. Full face

one finger moves down while the other is lifted up in rhythmic periods of fifty seconds.

Summary: This is very relaxing for the eyes and the face in general. It can relieve eye strain, which is valuable in this day and age with the increased use of electronic equipment.

Frontal Bone

Window: This is a beautiful hand position in which the index, middle, and ring fingers are making bilateral contact with the client's frontal bone, as shown in Figure 17.20.

Summary: Originally, the frontal bone had a suture in the middle above the nose and when the bone begins to breathe with PR, it feels as if a bird is flying. The sides of the frontal bone lift up like wings and then go back down.

Full Face

Window: This particular hand position, shown in Figure 17.21, is designed to sense the entire face breathing with PR. As with some of the previous facial hand positions, this hand position also gives a sense of a bird lifting off. Note that the practitioner's thumbs are over the ethmoid bone. It is important to sense the movement of the ethmoid bone in relationship to all the facial bones. This hand position and many others for the face are very beneficial for balancing the parasympathetic nervous system. The face is a parasympathetic organ.

Face in Sidelying

Some clients are not able to lie in the supine position for very long. As you can see in Figure 17.22, the practitioner's hands are supporting the client's face. The right hand is below the ear and left hand is above. Once again, the practitioner takes time to sense PR and allow the cranium to balance itself.

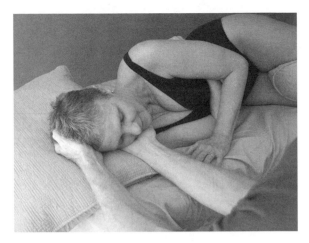

Figure 17.22. Face in sidelying

CHAPTER 18

The Cranial Vault and Base

Cranial Preparatory Window

As the practitioner prepares to make contact with the client's cranial vault or cranial base, I always recommend placing the hands lateral of the head, as seen in Figure 18.1. It is important to spend several minutes and imagine holding a large bowl of water that extends 15–20 inches off the client's skin. Then the practitioner can sense Primary Respiration (PR) breathing the bowl of water into his hands and back from the center of the client's cranium.

The practitioner slides his hands along the table toward the client's head until the little finger and hypothenar eminence make contact with the client's head underneath the ears. This is a nonspecific contact point to establish a basic palpatory relationship with the client's head. It is here where the practitioner, still imagining holding a bowl of water, begins a discovery process around the different activities and motions associated with the cranium if they present themselves.

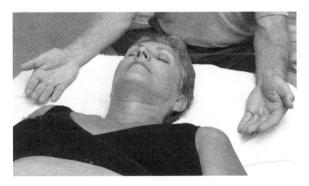

Figure 18.1. Cranial preparatory window

Parietal Lift

The parietal lift is perhaps one of the safest handholds that can be done with the client's cranium. It is the first of a two-part series of windows; the second window in the series is the temporal lift, described below. The basic exploration is to be able to decompress the tentorium in the cranium. The anatomy is quite precise. The tentorium has two leaves to it, a superior and inferior leaf (as mentioned in the previous chapter regarding the transverse sinus). The superior leaf has an attachment on the inferior lateral angles (ILAs) of the bilateral parietal bones.

199

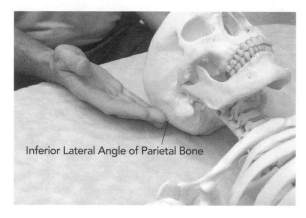

Inferior Lateral Angle of Parietal Bone

Figure 18.2. Parietal lift a

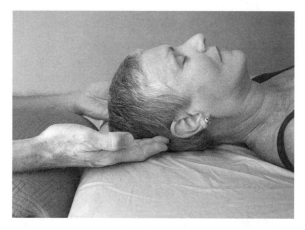

Figure 18.3. Parietal lift b

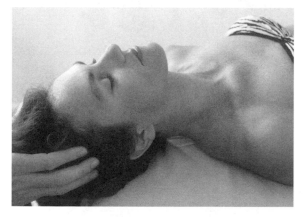

Figure 18.4. Parietal lift c

The inferior leaf has an attachment along the petrous ridge of the temporal bone. The majority of the twelve pairs of cranial nerves travel between these two leaves of the tentorium as the nerves exit the brain stem and traverse their various geographies to their end organs.

Window: Once the practitioner has synchronized his attention with the fluid body, he then solicits permission to make bilateral contact with the inferior lateral angle (ILA) of the client's parietal bones, as seen in Figures 18.2 and 18.3. Whenever first contact is made with the head, the practitioner solicits the comfort of the client. The anatomical position is quite precise and must be known by the practitioner.

Process: Now that proper contact has been established bilaterally with the ILAs of the client's parietal bones, the practitioner completes several cycles of attunement and notices the quality of motion present each time he brings his attention back to his hands.

Typically, the practitioner is only making contact with the client's ILAs with the pad of the middle finger of each hand. I like to say that this is a "one-fingered technique." It is important to use the pad of the finger rather than the tips. When the tips of the fingers are used, it creates too much flexion and compression, not only in the practitioner's hands, but possibly placing a compression into the client's cranium, brain, and nervous system.

Each time the practitioner brings his attention back to his finger pads, he is waiting for the various components of the cranial mechanism to reveal themselves in whatever sequence they choose. It is enough to just sense PR breathing in the fluid body three dimensionally from the ILAs.

Gradually, in clinical practice, the motion of the parietal bones and their relationship with the tentorium will manifest as a breathing motion much like the gull wings of the old DeLorean automobile and some Corvettes and Lamborghinis. The pivot point for the gull wing motion is more centrally located at the superior saggital suture of the cranium and in the breathing motion, the wings under the practitioner's finger pads flare out and the hinge below the superior saggital suture depresses. Then the motion reverses itself.

The practitioner may also shift the position of his hands to the parietal ridge bilaterally, as shown in Figure 18.4. From this position, the practitioner can sense the gull wing motion of the parietal bones and other movements of the cranium, such as the lateral fluctuation of the fluid body, the movement of the lateral ventricles, and even the neural tissue itself. It must be remembered that these are multiple levels of motion in the cranium (see Appendix) that appear in the practitioner's perception. Although these levels of motion are related to the layers of structure in the cranium, their appearance in a session is nonlinear.

After several cycles of observing this motion either at the ILAs or the parietal ridge, the parietal bones may move within the fluid matrix. The movement has a very clear sense of the parietal bones lifting bilaterally in a superior direction. In other words, since the practitioner is sitting at the top of the table, and consequently at the top of the client's head, it may feel as though the client's parietal bones are floating toward the practitioner's body. Their nature is to float in the direction of the practitioner's body and not retract back down. If they do retract back down, then just wait several more cycles until the bones are able to float on their own.

Summary: From a biodynamic perspective, the tentorium is actually an extension of the notochord embryologically. This means that the tentorium grew much like a sprout from the top of the notochord and spread out laterally. If the practitioner is willing to continue cycling through the attunement process with PR and not become overfocused on the cranium, holding the client's fluid body as a whole, the entire fluid body, brain, and heart of the client will have an opportunity to ignite biodynamically.

Temporal Lift

Window: The temporal lift is performed with stacked hands, as shown in Figure 18.5. This means that the practitioner places his right hand on top of the left hand and essentially cradles the client's occiput in the palm of the right hand (or the other dominant top hand) while the thumbs are free to sense the movement of the temporal bones via the mastoid tips.

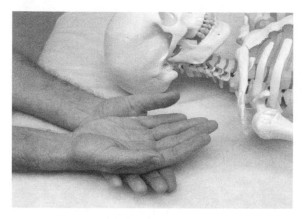

Figure 18.5. Temporal lift a

The temporal lift, which is used to evaluate the inferior leaf of the tentorium, is done with the thumbs under the mastoid processes bilaterally, as shown in Figures 18.6 and 18.7.

Once the practitioner has reoriented, resynchronized, and reattuned to PR and the natural world, any attention that is brought to the hands is done with the sense of holding a bowl of water and offering complete freedom for that bowl of water to breathe in all dimensions and directions.

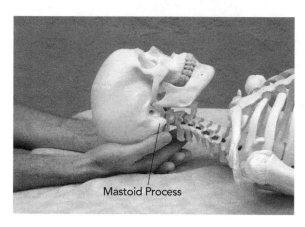

Mastoid Process

Figure 18.6. Temporal lift b

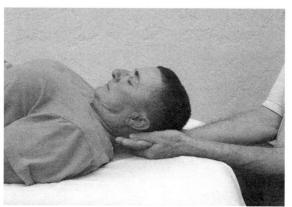

Figure 18.7. Temporal lift c
(with Valerie Gora)

Temporal Bones

The temporal bone is a highly sophisticated bone that houses the facial nerve, vestibular nerve, and acoustic nerve. These nerves generate important functions, especially associated with proprioception, somatic balance, and equilibrium. They also are associated with maintaining the head in an upright position with the eyes oriented to the horizon and the orienting reflex, as discussed in Chapter 17.

In addition, the temporomandibular joint (TMJ) is a part of the temporal bones. This bilateral joint is extremely sensitive to forces coming from the face and the function of eating and swallowing. Mandibular whiplash is a common side effect of motor vehicle accidents. This occurs when the mandible dislocates from the TMJ, which may result in damage to the TMJ and subsequent trauma to the temporal bones. Consequently, the temporal lift requires that the practitioner understand the bilateral motion dynamics of the TMJ, the motions of the temporal bones, and the flexion and extension movement of the tentorium itself. This adds additional dimensions and layers of experience to the practitioner's perception of Primary Respiration. These movements occur three dimensionally as one unified dynamic and thus caution must be used when isolating aspects of the total movement pattern.

Window: This is a bilateral contact with the practitioner's thumbs directly on the mastoid processes of the temporal bones, as shown in Figure 18.8.

In Figure 18.9, I clearly show both of the thumbs in position over the mastoid processes.

In Figure 18.10, you can see the right hand in position on the client's temporal bone. The thumb fits snugly under the client's ear. The rest of the fingers simply rest wherever they land. The intention is to sense the external and internal rotation of the temporal bones. This occurs both through the motion of the temporal squama and mastoid process.

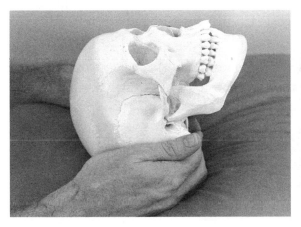

Figure 18.8. Temporal bones a

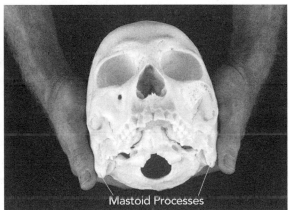

Figure 18.9. Temporal bones b

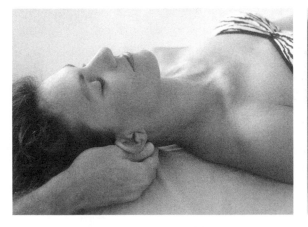

Figure 18.10. Temporal bones c

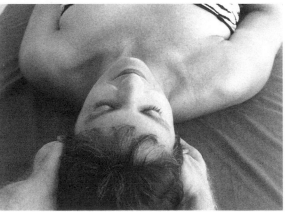

Figure 18.11. Temporal bones d

In Figure 18.11, the hands have a bilateral contact with the client's temporal bones. This is a great place to listen more directly to the fluid fields of the cranial base and how they breathe with PR.

The motion of the temporal bones may feel like a figure eight motion. In addition, it is not unusual for the temporal bones to stillpoint at the end phase of their expansion cycle. Traditionally, this was called an EV4 (expansion of the fourth ventricle). The practitioner would know that the temporal bones were in their end point of external rotation because the bilateral mastoid processes were moving medially and posteriorly while the temporal squama moved laterally. Thus it was easy to simply hold the mastoid processes in and down as long as the contact over the temporal squama allowed for external rotation.

The temporal bones seek to balance themselves by going through phases of stillpoint and motion synchronized with PR. I typically will wait for a stillpoint, especially if there is any history of head trauma, particularly one or more concussions. This is a wonderful hand position for any client who has a history of head concussions. I believe it is possible to delay or prevent chronic traumatic encephalopathy (CTE). This is a relatively new diagnosis in the field of concussions, referring to those clients who have received repeated concussions, such as football players. The temporal bones will feel like they are moving in glue. It is very important to synchronize with PR to allow the fluid body to heal itself around the brain.

Summary: Traditionally, it was taught that the temporal bones would stillpoint at the end of their phase of external rotation. From a biodynamic point of view, this may or may not happen, according to the intentions of PR.

Traditional Vault Hold

Regarding the sphenobasilar (SBJ) joint space, I have gone through an evolution of several different hand positions for it. The first hand position is, of course, the traditional Sutherland vault hold, shown in Figures 18.12, 18.13, 18.14, and 18.15.

Figures 18.12 and 18.13 show two variations for the location of the practitioner's thumbs. Figure 18.12 shows the thumbs overlapping and Figure 18.13 shows the thumbs straddling each other with the hands making more of a full-contoured contact with the client's cranium. The position of the thumbs will be determined by the size of the practitioner's hands and the size of the client's head.

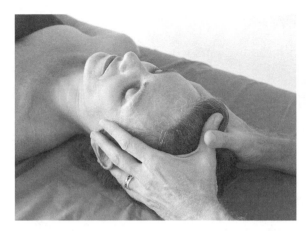

Figure 18.12. Traditional vault hold a

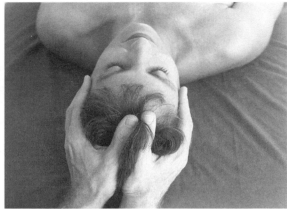

Figure 18.13. Traditional vault hold b

Figures 18.14 and 18.15 show the following: The pads of the index fingers are on the greater wings of the sphenoid bone. The pads of the middle fingers are over the TMJ and masseter muscle. The pads of the ring fingers are under the ears. The pads of the little fingers are in contact with the occiput.

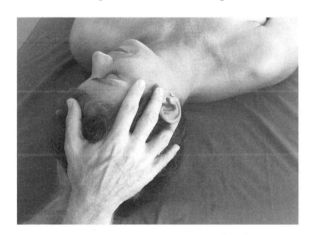

Figure 18.14. Traditional vault hold c

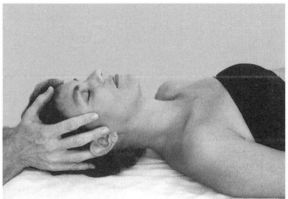

Figure 18.15. Traditional vault hold d

Process: The challenge with the traditional vault hold is the different sizes of practitioner's hands. The most important contact is with the greater wings of the sphenoid and if the practitioner's hands are not large, the contact with the temporal bones and occiput may strain the hands or be impossible to do. Consequently, the Becker hold, described below, is the best alternative. Alternatively, a simple thumb position for decompressing the sphenoid can be explored.

Sphenoid Decompression

I periodically use this window with some clients who have experienced severe head trauma.

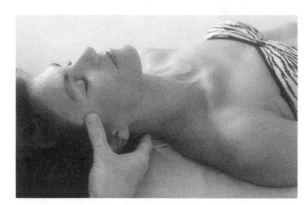

Figure 18.16. Sphenoid decompression

Window: The practitioner places the pads of the thumbs bilaterally on the greater wings and the ring and pinkies around the occiput, as shown in Figure 18.16. The thumbs get a better mechanical contact on the greater wings for a lift toward the ceiling.

Becker Hold

The Becker hold is used to transition into biodynamic practice when contacting the cranial base and synchronizing with PR. In this window, the practitioner simply listens for the activity of the two metabolic fields that form the cranial base embryonically. The cranial base is made from the tip of the notochord, which becomes basiocciput and basisphenoid, as shown in Figure 18.17. The metabolic fields in question involve a three-dimensional expansion and contraction from the tip of the notochord or, in the case of the adult, the actual SBJ itself moving at the rate of PR.

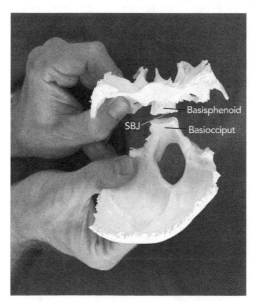

Figure 18.17. Becker hold a

The second metabolic field that forms the cranial base is a longitudinal motion perceived by the hands, much like holding a tunnel or two moving longitudinally and back between the third ventricle and the coccyx at the rate of PR. This particular window is a variation on the classical Sutherland vault hold. Over the past several decades the traditional vault hold has changed into a hand position that was used by Dr. Rollin Becker in his career. It was then subsequently taught as an alternative vault hold.

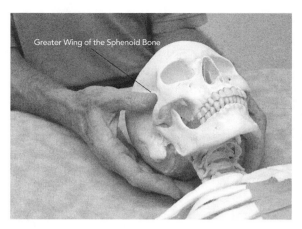

Figure 18.18. Becker hold b

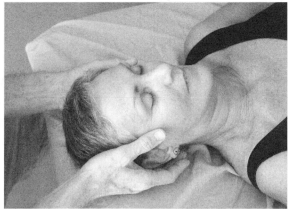

Figure 18.19. Becker hold c

Window: This is a bilateral hand position with contact on the client's greater wings of the sphenoid bone and lateral masses of the occipital bone, as seen in Figure 18.18.

As with any hand position around the head, the practitioner, while seated above the client's head, places his hands six inches laterally of the client's ears and begins to imagine holding a bowl of water and sensing PR.

Once the practitioner has synchronized attention with PR, both in himself and around the client's head, the practitioner negotiates verbal permission to make contact with the side of the client's face.

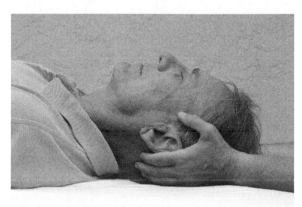

Figure 18.20. Becker hold d
(with Valerie Gora's hands)

The sides of the thumbs are placed buoyantly over the skin covering the greater wings of the sphenoid, as shown in Figure 18.19.

The palms of the practitioner's hands are over the ears, but not in contact with the client's ears, if possible. Figure 18.20 shows a variation with a practitioner whose hands are small in relation to a large cranium.

The practitioner uses the little fingers bilaterally to find the occiput right where it meets the table.

This particular window requires that the wrist and forearms of the practitioner be supported very securely.

Occiput CV4 (Compression of the Fourth Ventricle)

The traditional starting point to settle the whole body and nervous system is called the CV4 (compression of the fourth ventricle). As Dr. Becker said, this area has the most common sutural fixation from a vaginal birth that persists into adulthood. This is because there are important relationships between the occipitomastoid suture and the fourth ventricle, the jugular vein, and the ninth, tenth, and eleventh cranial nerves. The CV4 is birth work.

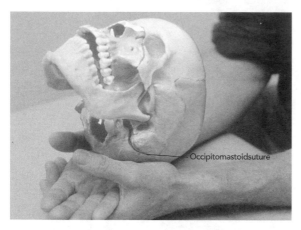

Figure 18.21. Occiput CV4 a
(photographed by Robert Cutter)

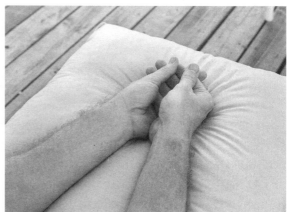

Figure 18.22. Occiput CV4 b

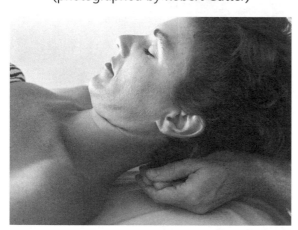

Figure 18.23. Occiput CV4 c

Window: The palpation is done with the thenar eminences at the base of the thumbs of the practitioner. The thenar eminences are placed bilaterally on the squamous portion of the client's occiput, as shown in Figure 18.21. It is here where the occiput itself has its greatest range of motion just medial to the occipito-mastoid suture.

The hands are stacked as shown in Figure 18.22. I typically use my dominant hand as the top hand in the stack.

The practitioner evaluates the movement of the occipitomastoid suture and its continuity with the occipitopetrous suture by using the hand position of the traditional CV4. The thenar eminences at the base of the thumbs are supporting the head of the client, as shown in Figure 18.23.

The practitioner lifts the client's head and may ask the client to seat it comfortably in his hands once in position. Sometimes a millimeter of movement can make this hand position extremely comfortable or uncomfortable. The practitioner also wants to make sure the hands are not pulling the client's hair.

Process: There are some important nuances with the location and activity of the practitioner's hands. When the side of the client's occipitomastoid suture that is restricted has been identified, the intention is to allow a gentle CV4. There will be a very slight amount of extra contact coming from the practitioner's hand on the side of the restriction. This is not a direct medial compression. Otherwise, the opposite hand would have to respond with an equal amount of compression or the client's head would rotate off of the midline and off the practitioner's hands.

Consequently, the hand that is offering the extra contact is gently rolling medially with its thenar eminence. It is micro movement. The rolling motion is coming from the thenar eminence at the base of the thumb. This offers a very gentle traction to open the occipitomastoid suture. As with a traditional CV4, when the occiput has reached an end point of medial motion, the practitioner holds and balances the occiput in that position until the potency builds (2–3 CPM) in the fourth ventricle and pushes the hands out.

Another nuance with the hands is important here. While the occiput is being held in a medial position, I like to use my thenar eminences of both hands to gently invite a figure eight motion into the squama of the occiput while I am waiting for the potency to build in the fourth ventricle. This rolling and alternating decompressing-compressing dynamic is done very briefly and subtly in the tempo of PR. The majority of exploration is about listening and waiting for PR to build potency in the ventricles for ignition. It is not unusual to track the lateral expansion of the occiput several times after it has pushed out in order to get a more complete normalization of movement through the suture and the fluid fields. It is not advisable to compress the occiput this way, even with a very slight compression, more than two times in the session.

Igniting the Bird in the Ventricles

Figure 18.24 is a drawing that Josefine Frind, an assistant of mine, made in Germany some years ago. The outline of the ventricles can be seen as a kind of watermark in the whole figure of the bird. Please keep this image in mind while you are practicing. This exploration requires concentration on orienting, synchronizing, and attuning.

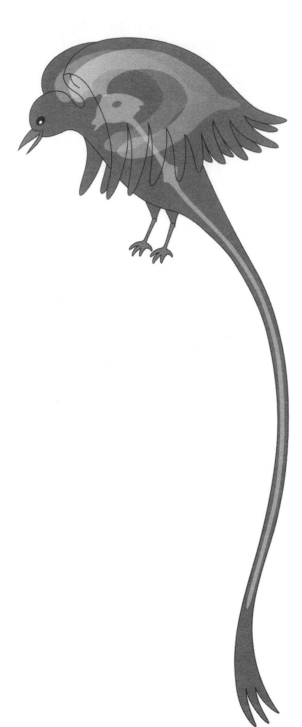

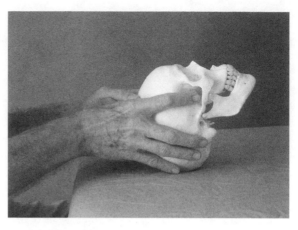

Figure 18.25. Igniting the bird a

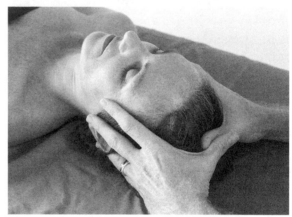

Figure 18.26. Igniting the bird b

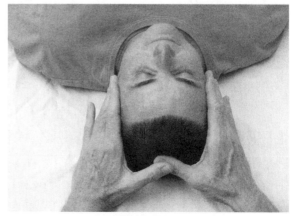

Figure 18.24. The bird in the ventricles (image by Josefine Frind, reprinted with permission)

Figure 18.27. Igniting the bird c (with Valerie Gora)

Window: Client is supine. Practitioner is sitting at the head of the table and rests attention in his third ventricle and central stillness at the beginning and then occasionally through the exploration.

The practitioner negotiates permission to make contact with the pads of his index and middle fingers bilaterally on the greater wings of the sphenoid. The lengths of the index fingers are positioned along the coronal suture, as shown in Figure 18.25, and the thumbs are positioned around or on top of bregma, as shown in Figures 18.26 and 18.27.

Regarding the hand position, the most important contact is over bregma with the pads of the thumbs as they are either crossed on top of one another or the tips touching one another, depending on the size of the practitioner's hands. NO pressure is placed on bregma. It is a buoyant touch with a focus on the backs of the hands.

Process: The practitioner synchronizes his attention with PR in the client's fluid body and then the cranium. The greater wings of the sphenoid will tend to move laterally for fifty seconds while bregma depresses inferiorly for fifty seconds. Then the cycle reverses itself. The perception of this motion must be precise. These are the wings of the bird in the lateral and central ventricles expressing themselves.

Bregma may begin to feel as if it is breathing on a line down through the third and fourth ventricles.

Gradually, Primary Respiration will express itself more fully and there may be a sense or an image of a bird in flight. An image of a particular bird may appear to the practitioner.

Following this hand position, the sacrum and feet must be contacted and the whole fluid body of the client allowed to amplify with PR. This includes checking the longitudinal fluctuation.

Summary: This is a powerful exploration that I only recommend trying after the third session with a client. It has the potential to recalibrate the neuroendocrine immune axis between the pineal gland in the posterior third ventricle and the pituitary gland in the anterior third ventricle. It should only be attempted once in any session. Time must be given to rebalance the fluid body as necessary afterward.

CHAPTER 19

Anterior Midline

The anterior midline is an embryological seam from bregma to the pubic symphysis. It represents the last phase of closure over the ventral surface of the body, which does not take place until several months after birth. It actually does not close physically until a month after birth when the umbilicus has healed from cutting the umbilical cord.

Eight windows are described in the Process paragraphs below. The windows are:

- Bregma to intraorbital ligament (IL) (Figures 19.1 and 19.2)
- IL to upper lip (philtrum) (Figures 19.3 and 19.4)
- Philtrum to mid mandible (mentalis) (Figures 19.5 and 19.6)
- Mentalis to sternoclavicular notch (SCN) (Figures 19.7 and 19.8)
- SCN to xyphoid process (XP) (Figures 19.9 and 19.10)
- XP to umbilicus (Figures 19.11 and 19.12)
- Umbilicus to pubis (Figures 19.13 and 19.14)
- Finally, the Pietà or feet or both

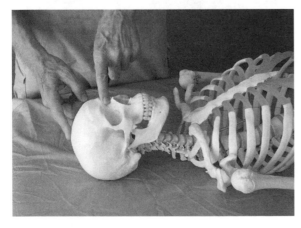

Figure 19.1. Anterior midline a

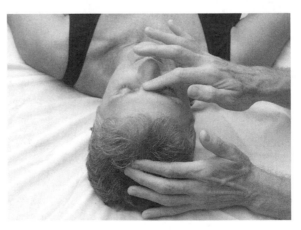

Figure 19.2. Anterior midline b

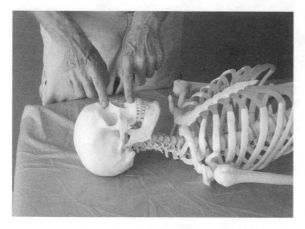

Figure 19.3. Anterior midline c

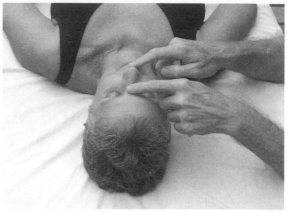

Figure 19.4. Anterior midline d

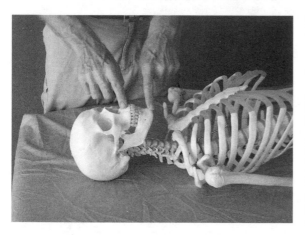

Figure 19.5. Anterior midline e

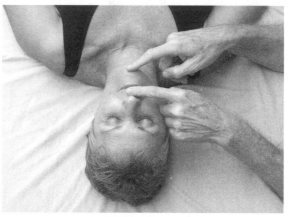

Figure 19.6. Anterior midline f

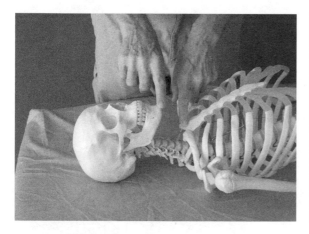

Figure 19.7. Anterior midline g

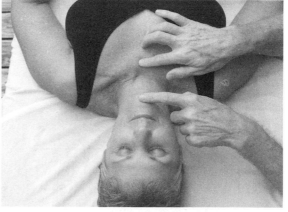

Figure 19.8. Anterior midline h

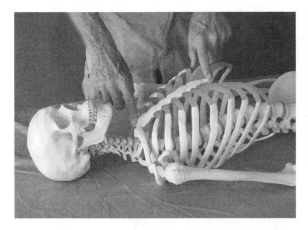

Figure 19.9. Anterior midline i

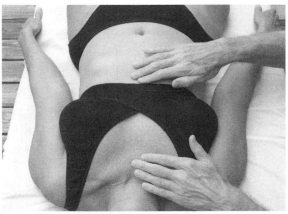

Figure 19.10. Anterior midline j

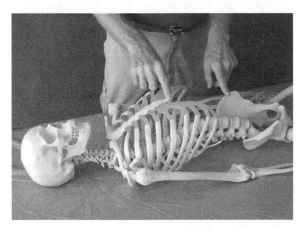

Figure 19.11. Anterior midline k

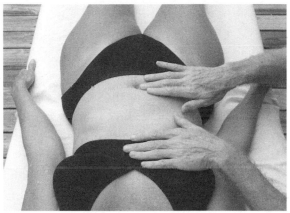

Figure 19.12. Anterior midline l

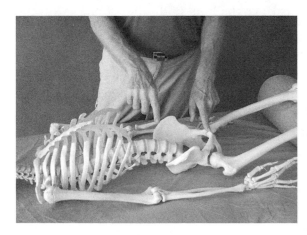

Figure 19.13. Anterior midline m

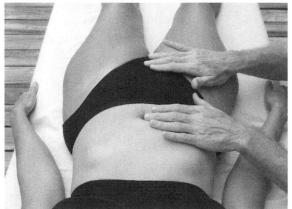

Figure 19.14. Anterior midline n

Process: Orient to 3D stillness. Synchronize with 3D heart and blood. Let the fluid body decompress along the seam.

For each window, sense each of the two points connecting via Primary Respiration (PR) and then all the way posteriorly to the spine.

For each position, the practitioner overlaps her fingers or leapfrogs over the lower hand such that one finger remains on the lower point of the previous pair of points while the other finger is moving.

The *first* finger contact is on bregma and the intraorbital ligament, sensing PR.

The *second* finger placement is on the intraorbital ligament and philtrum. Once again the focus is on sensing PR in any dimension.

The *third* finger placement is on the philtrum and the mentalis of the mandible. The mentalis was originally a suture dividing the mandible into two portions.

The *fourth* finger placement is on the mentalis and the sternoclavicular notch.

The *fifth* finger placement is on the sternoclavicular notch and the xyphoid process at the bottom of the sternum.

The *sixth* finger placement is on the xyphoid process and the umbilicus. In the photo, for the sake of the reader being able to see the umbilicus, I have moved my middle finger of my right hand slightly lateral of the umbilicus. Normally, the finger would be over the umbilicus.

The *seventh* finger placement is over the umbilicus and the pubic symphysis. This is the last hand position for the anterior midline.

It is recommended that the practitioner make contact with the client in the Pietà position, feet, or sacrum to balance the fluid body after contact with the anterior midline.

Summary: If the practitioner does not know where the pubic symphysis is located in the client, she should have the client show where it is located. All of these hand positions involve sensing PR. I am frequently asked if the entire sequence needs to be done each time the anterior midline is approached. The answer is no, but it is important to practice all of them periodically in order to differentiate when it is appropriate to use all or some of the hand positions for the anterior midline.

Sometimes I go through this process while I am seated at the side of the client and other times I will do it standing. It does not make a lot of difference, except that in both cases, the arms need to have stable support.

CHAPTER 20

Ready Reference to Photographs

Chapter 13: Preliminary Instructions and First Contact

Figure 13.1. Pietà a (skeleton) This is a photo with my hands in the position I call the Pietà. One hand is under the knee or it can be slightly above the knee. My superior hand is gently around the top of the shoulder. It is important to not have the superior hand lifting or supporting the scapula. It is simply around the deltoid muscle and possibly touching the superior border of the scapula. The intention is to sense Primary Respiration from the fluid body of the client breathing as one whole movement into both hands.

Figure 13.2. Pietà b This shows the position of my hands on a client. Please notice my superior hand is not lifting the shoulder at all, but simply cradling the upper arm and top of the shoulder. I like to sense Primary Respiration coming from the whole fluid body of the client into both of my hands. I also like to move my attention to my heart and sense Primary Respiration coming from the client with my sternum, rib cage, and heart.

Figure 13.3. Feet Here I am holding the client's feet. The weight of the heels is in the palms of my hands. I like to begin with this position or the Pietà. With both positions, I can concentrate on my posture and make sure I am oriented to a base of quietness in my body. Holding the feet like this and at the side and on the dorsal surface of the feet as other practitioners do are all good positions. It begins allowing the autonomic nervous system of the client to settle.

Chapter 14: Lower Extremities Supine

Figure 14.1. Cuboid-navicular a (skeleton with labels) This image shows my index fingers making contact with the ventral surface of the cuboid and navicular bones. The cuboid-navicular joint space is considered to be an analog of the sphenobasilar joint space.

217

Figure 14.2. Cuboid-navicular b (skeleton with labels) This image shows my thumbs on the dorsal surface of the cuboid and navicular bones. I always image the client as whole, no matter what the location of my hands.

Figure 14.3. Cuboid-navicular c Here you can see my hand contact with my client's foot. Please note that I changed the angle of my arms in order to accommodate a better view of the position of my thumbs and index finger. Normally, the practitioner's arms are going to be parallel to the top of the table. This is a wonderful way to approach the whole body through this joint space in the feet. Not only can you balance the foot and its connection with the ground, but it also helps to stabilize all the diaphragms of the body up through the cranium.

Figure 14.4. Legs supine a (skeleton with labels) This image shows my hands supporting the tibia and fibula. I like to get my thumbs close to the head of the fibula and lateral malleoli.

Figure 14.5. Legs supine b This image shows how to support the client's leg. The intention of this particular hand position and the whole exploration of the lower extremities in general is to disengage the fight-flight component of the sympathetic nervous system in the client. Fight-flight is usually held in the neurovascular bundle and interosseous membrane between the tibia and fibula. I wait for Primary Respiration to begin thawing out the interosseous membrane and for the tibia and fibula to begin to breathe with Primary Respiration in the whole.

Figure 14.6. Legs supine c Here you can see the same hand position. This time my thumbs are clearly visible on the lateral malleoli and close to the head of the fibula.

Figure 14.7. Legs supine d (skeleton with labels) This image shows my lower hand under the knee and my upper hand with the tips of the fingers making contact with the spinous processes of the lumbar vertebra.

Figure 14.8. Legs supine e This image shows my hand position under the client. Once I have begun to sense Primary Respiration moving through the interosseous membrane between the tibia and fibula, I switch one hand to the underside of the knee and the other hand to contact with the lumbar vertebra. The intention is to be able to sense Primary Respiration connecting the lower extremity through to the lower lumbar vertebra.

Figure 14.9. Lower extremity in sidelying a (skeleton with labels) This next lower-extremity exploration is valuable for clients who cannot lie supine for too long. The client is in sidelying, which allows specific contact with the lateral malleoli and head of the fibula. Please note that the index finger and thumb are together as if I were plucking a tissue from a box of Kleenex. It is easier to sense Primary Respiration this way.

Figure 14.10. Lower extremity in sidelying b Here you can see how I use my fingertips to make contact with the client's fibula. The intention is to feel how Primary Respiration breathes the fibula. This is called intraosseous motion. Sometimes, the fibula will torsion slowly and then shorten and lengthen slowly. These are its embryonic growth patterns.

Figure 14.11. Lower extremity in sidelying c (skeleton with labels) This image shows the next position with contact over the greater trochanter of the femur and the pad of my index finger of my lower hand will be on the midline just below the patella.

Figure 14.12. Lower extremity in sidelying d My top hand is over the greater trochanter in a tissue-plucking position. My bottom hand, however, shows the pad of my middle finger inferior to the patella. Either the index or middle finger is fine. The intention is to sense Primary Respiration breathing the femur intraosseously. The femur holds a lot of stress and may take some time for it to fully resuscitate with Primary Respiration.

Figure 14.13. Lower extremity in sidelying e (skeleton) Here you can see my hands slightly exaggerated with the thumbs over the greater trochanter and my fingers spread over the crest of the ilium.

Figure 14.14. Lower extremity in sidelying f My hands are positioned over the client's greater trochanter and the crest of the ilium. I typically work with my clients clothed; consequently, I ask permission for my left arm (as in this photo) to rest on the leg of the client. It is important to have as much support for the wrists, arms, and elbows as possible whenever treating the client. The intention here is to sense the entire hip bone breathing with Primary Respiration. With the fulcrum being the greater trochanter, the hip bone tends to have a gull-wing type of lifting and closing motion, similar to that of the DeLorean car. It is important to wait until the entire circumference of the bone around to the front at the pubic symphysis and inferiorly to the ischial tuberosity is behaving as one whole gull wing. Please refer to Figure 14.15 for an image of the hip bone.

Figure 14.15. Embryological derivatives of the innominate bone (skeleton with labels) This is an image of the three embryological derivatives of the innominate bone. They are: the ischium, which is the bottom left portion of the bone; the ilium, which is its largest part above the acetabular fossa; and the pubic bone, which is the bottom right portion of the bone as it is viewed here. Please note that all three bones have their fulcrum in the center of the acetabular fossa of the innominate bone. Thus when the practitioner has his thumbs crossed over the greater trochanter, he is able to sense these three derivatives like a trifold gull wing lifting up and down and the two fossae of the innominate bone breathing toward and away from each other. In addition, an axle between the two fossae of the innominate bone breathes with Primary Respiration on the horizontal axis between the fossae.

Figure 14.16. Lower extremity in sidelying g (skeleton with labels) My thumbs are making contact with the coccyx and second sacral segment of the sacrum.

Figure 14.17. Lower extremity in sidelying h Here you can see how my hands make contact with the sacrum, although in this photo, my thumbs are closer together than in the previous photo with the skeleton. Both positions are correct. The rest of my fingers are spread out over the hip and gluteal area of my client. The intention is to sense Primary Respiration breathing the sacrum in conjunction with the hip bone breathing as well.

Chapter 15: Abdomen and Pelvis

Figure 15.1. Umbilicus a This is an image of the client's abdomen. I frequently invite students to draw the different directions that the viscera make directly on this image.

Figure 15.2. Umbilicus b Here my hands are located one above the umbilicus and one below. The intention here is to sense the developmental movements of the midgut that include the small and large intestines. The intestines make a spiral movement up and out of the abdomen and back down and in, following their embryonic pattern with Primary Respiration.

Figure 15.3. Umbilicus c Here the client is prone and my hands are located above and below the umbilicus. This position is beneficial for sensing how the hands and arms mimic the umbilical vein and artery coming from the placenta. This is sensed as the movement of Primary Respiration coming from the heart of the practitioner through the arms and hands into the client's umbilical area and then back. This also can balance the respiratory and pelvic diaphragms.

Figure 15.4. Sacrum a (skeleton) This image shows a model of the sacrum superimposed on top of the client's actual sacrum in prone position.

Figure 15.5. Sacrum b The client here is in prone position being supported with a head rest. I am making very light buoyant contact to sense the motion of the sacrum. This image is just to see the location of the sacrum in relationship to my hand.

Figure 15.6. Sacrum c (skeleton) Here my hands are making contact with the remnants of the primitive streak in the sacrum. The middle finger of my right hand is around the coccyx. The ring finger and little finger of my left hand are on the first and second sacral segment.

Figure 15.7. Sacrum d (skeleton) Here I have superimposed a model of a sacrum with the client supine. My hands are in position to make contact with the primitive streak. The intention is to connect with the sacrum breathing with Primary Respiration, as well as the whole pelvis and gradually the entire fluid body of the client.

Figure 15.8. Sacrum e My left hand approaches the client from just below the gluteal fold. Sometimes, I ask the client to bend her knee in order to make it easier to find the bottom of the sacrum and the coccyx. My top hand is approaching the base of the sacrum from slightly above the crest of the ilium.

Figure 15.9. Liver a (skeleton) This hand position is for contacting the liver. My right hand is under the floating ribs and my top hand is spanning the edge of the costal arch. The middle finger of my left hand is pointing toward the middle to upper left arm of the client.

Figure 15.10. Liver b Notice how my left arm is propped up with a pillow. This is very important. The intention is to sense the liver breathing with Primary Respiration, like a bellows that is moving slowly toward the cardia (space where the esophagus enters the stomach as it passes through the diaphragm) and back.

Figure 15.11. Liver c Sometimes I like to cradle the entire liver in order to sense its faster motility as it moves toward the umbilicus and back. The liver needs to be checked in almost all clients. Metabolic syndrome, insulin resistance, obesity, hepatitis, and many other problems reside in the liver.

Figure 15.12. Bladder a (skeleton with labels) This image shows the heel of my hand making contact with the pubic symphysis of the skeleton. The bladder is located directly underneath the pubic bone and thus this is the starting position for sensing the bladder and its motion.

Figure 15.13. Bladder b I have my hand positioned on the client's abdomen with the heel of my hand on the pubic symphysis. Primary Respiration reveals the motion of the bladder and the touch needs to be very, very buoyant. The bladder has a very slow rocking motion and will come to a stillpoint and then deepen into Primary Respiration. The bladder is vitally important as it is the main structural support organ of the pelvic floor. In other words, all the organs in the pelvis have suspensory ligaments anchored to the bladder.

Figure 15.14. Small intestine Here my hands are close together and lateral of the umbilicus in order to sense the motility of the small intestine. The small intestine moves like a pair of windshield wipers. Thus each hand has one windshield washer. It is important to balance both the small and large intestines together. If the practitioner shifts his attention to Primary Respiration then the developmental movements of the midgut become apparent.

Figure 15.15. Large intestine Here my hands are located lateral of the umbilicus. My fingertips are pointing superiorly. This position is used to sense the faster functional movement (motility) of the large intestine as it rotates clockwise and counterclockwise. Remember that the ascending colon is located just below the surface of the abdominal muscles and thus quite easy to palpate.

Figure 15.16. Diaphragms a (skeleton with labels) This is a very valuable way to hold the respiratory and pelvic diaphragms. I have the tip of my finger under the coccyx and my other hand under the floating ribs of the skeleton. It is possible to have your fingers either make contact with the spinous processes of the vertebra or even be underneath them. The key here is comfort and ease.

Figure 15.17. Diaphragms b Here I have my hands in the same location except on the opposite side of the body. The intention here is to sense diaphragmatic breathing as it fills both hands during the inhalation and exhalation cycle. Gradually, the practitioner wants to become aware of the relationship of diaphragmatic breathing to Primary Respiration. While paying attention to the client's breathing, it is important for the practitioner to have awareness of his own breathing periodically.

Figure 15.18. Kidneys Here I have my hands on the kidneys bilaterally. The client is prone and her head is supported in a head rest. It is important to discover how the kidneys move with Primary Respiration. The embryonic kidneys go all the way up to the neck and the adult kidneys expand and contract with Primary Respiration on a vector toward the heart and away from the heart.

Figure 15.19. Hip bones supine a (skeleton with labels) Here my hands are supporting the entire hip bone. The top hand has contact with the anterior superior iliac spine. The bottom hand has contact with the ischial tuberosity. The fingers do not need to be under the tuberosity, but merely touching it from the side.

Figure 15.20. Hip bones supine b Sometimes, you need to ask the client to lift the hip up in order to make contact with the tuberosity underneath.

Figure 15.21. Hip bones supine c Here you can see the contact with my bottom hand resting on the table. It is very important that the top hand be propped under the elbow with a pillow, which cannot be seen in this photo. In addition, my body is turned and looking diagonally toward the opposite leg and foot of the client.

Figure 15.22. Hip in flexion a (skeleton with labels) This photo shows my hands making bilateral contact with both ischial tuberosities. The knees of the client need to be flexed. Because of the size of my hands, I am able to also make contact with the greater trochanter.

Figure 15.23. Hip in flexion b This perspective shows my hands in position on a client with her knees flexed.

Figure 15.24. Hip in flexion c This view shows portions of both of my hands on the client's hips. Her knees are flexed and together. The client needs to have his or her feet splayed out laterally in order to have the knees rest together. This is a wonderful way to balance the hips and pelvic floor, especially for a pregnant woman.

Chapter 16: The Spine, Trunk, and Neck

Figure 16.1. Snake a (skeleton with labels) Here my hands are making contact with the lower thoracic spine and the upper lumbar spine. The spinous processes of the vertebra are resting in the palm of my hand. Sometimes it is uncomfortable for a practitioner to have his hands together and it is okay to spread the hands to find the maximum amount of comfort necessary to sit and listen to the spine.

Figure 16.2. Snake b Here my hands are oriented to the thoracic spine. The hands can be placed on any part of the spine in order to sense Primary Respiration moving up and down the spine. I frequently choose the thoracic spine to sense the relationship of breathing to the spine, especially for any client who spends a lot of time in front of a computer. Gradually with Primary Respiration, the spine will soften and synchronize with the motion of the respiratory diaphragm.

Figure 16.3. Lungs (skeleton) Here I have my hands bilaterally on the costal arch of the ribs. This is the way I like to sense Primary Respiration moving the lungs. Primary Respiration breathes the lungs toward its original point between the third and fifth cervical vertebra. This is where the lungs originated in the embryo. From the vantage point of the costal arch, I can sense Primary Respiration breathing the lungs back and forth from the lower cervical spine. I like to either stand for this hand position or sit on the edge of the treatment table.

Figure 16.4. Notochord a The client is sidelying and I use the backs of my hands to contact the sacrum and the occiput. From this position, I like to sense Primary Respiration on its longitudinal axis and simply let the spine breathe.

Figure 16.5. Notochord b (skeleton with labels) This image shows the relationship of the occiput to the sacrum. Some texts have called this the core link, indicating the attachment that the dura mater has on the foramen magnum of the occiput and the second sacral segment.

Figure 16.6. Bilateral shoulders Here I have my hands on the client's shoulders. Before I make any contact with a client's neck and head, I always make contact around the shoulders or clavicles. In this case, my hands are gently cupping the upper arm bilaterally. I simply settle and sense Primary Respiration. I also like to bring attention to my own heart and sense the client's Primary Respiration coming from her midline as it pushes and pulls against my trunk and heart.

Figure 16.7. Ipsilateral shoulder a (skeleton) Here I am making contact with the shoulder ipsilaterally. My lower hand is under the scapula, as you can see. My top hand has contact over the upper arm with my middle finger touching the clavicle.

Figure 16.8. Ipsilateral shoulder b Here my hands are on the client and the intention is to sense Primary Respiration breathing the arm, shoulder, trunk, and neck as one single continuum.

Figure 16.9. Clavicles a (skeleton) This image shows the pads of my fingers spread out around the mid to distal end of the clavicles bilaterally. The reader can see that there are several options for making contact with the clavicles depending on a client's history and the individual treatment progression.

Figure 16.10. Clavicles b Here I have my fingers on the client's clavicles. Once again, I would like to stress the importance of making sure the practitioner is not exhaling on the client's face. I also want to have practitioners focus on sensing Primary Respiration moving back and forth from the client's midline with the sternum, heart, and trunk. Frequently, in this hand position, the index fingers and thumbs of both hands form a type of a yoke around the thoracic inlet. This is a convenient location to sense Primary Respiration as a tunnel moving back and forth between the yoke of the practitioner's hands.

Figure 16.11. Clavicles c (skeleton) In this image, I am making contact with the proximal and distal end of the right clavicle. I am using the pads of my fingertips. When a client has had a broken clavicle or other trauma to that area in which the fascia of the clavicles has tightened, this is a wonderful way to sense Primary Respiration repairing the clavicle.

Figure 16.12. Clavicles d (skeleton) There are several ways to make contact with the clavicles. Here I am making bilateral contact with the clavicles with my index finger and thumb in the "tissue plucking" position. This is one way to sense Primary Respiration moving through the clavicles from proximal to distal. It is also a good way to sense the clavicles rotating back and forth.

Figure 16.13. Clavicles e Here my fingers are on the client's clavicles in the tissue-plucking position. Once again, you can see how my arm is being propped with a pillow. This is a very gentle way to make contact with the clavicles to get specific information about how they breathe with Primary Respiration. Always allow the hands to accommodate to the rise and fall of the trunk in breathing.

Figure 16.14. Pleura This hand position is for contacting the cervical pleural ligament. It is the originating point of the lungs and, in the adult, the pleura is suspended from the cervical spine as high up as the third cervical vertebra. Here my fingers are located by the transverse processes of the mid to lower cervical spine. I like to wait and just sense all the tissues melting with Primary Respiration. Gradually, the client's breathing will expand the upper lobes of the lungs and consequently the pleura, which can be readily sensed with the fingers.

Figure 16.15. Heart fulcrum a (skeleton) This next series of hand positions is called the heart fulcrum. The embryonic heart arises around the third cervical vertebra. Here you can see my hands with the fingertips together around the middle of the neck. Obviously, the hands go under the neck (not on top, as shown in the photo, for viewing the finger position).

Figure 16.16. Heart fulcrum b (skeleton) Here my hands and fingers are under the neck in the correct position for sensing the heart fulcrum.

Figure 16.17. Heart fulcrum c The intention of this hand position is to be able to sense how Primary Respiration breathes in an anterior to posterior dimension. As I tune into Primary Respiration, very gradually, I sense the pads of my fingertips lifting up and gradually being let back down by Primary Respiration. This is a wonderful way to balance the space above and below the foramen magnum.

Figure 16.18. Scapular EV4 a (skeleton) This skill is called a scapular EV4. Here my hands are located under the scapula bilaterally. I am listening to the whole fluid body breathe and waiting for it to stillpoint at the end of its expansion phase, thus the term EV4. Formerly, EV4 referred to the stillpoint at the end of the expansion of the fourth ventricle. Here the term is applied biodynamically to the entire fluid body at the level of the scapula.

Figure 16.19. Scapular EV4 b Here you can see my hands located under the client's scapula. Not only is it possible to sense the whole fluid body from this position, but also the heart. I will frequently visualize the embryonic heart as if it were filling the entire thoracic cavity. Then I sense the heart breathing with Primary Respiration.

Figure 16.20. Scapular EV4 c This image is a lateral view of my hands under the client's scapula. It is a personal preference whether the practitioner supports the entire scapula with the fingers or with the palms of the hands. I frequently use the palms of my hands to support the whole scapula.

Figure 16.21. Arms and hands a (skeleton) This sequence on the upper extremity begins with holding the hand and supporting the elbow in the palm of my other hand. Please note the position of my thumb and the thumb of the skeleton.

Figure 16.22. Arms and hands b Here you can see the same hand position on the client except I am using her left arm. It is important to motion test the arm with a very slight motion to make sure no tension is being held in the arm. The total weight of the arm is in my hands. The intention here is to sense Primary Respiration breathing along the long axis of the bones of the forearm.

Figure 16.23. Arms and hands c (skeleton) Once I sense Primary Respiration breathing in the hand and forearm of the client, I then shift the hand that was under the elbow to a position where my fingertips make contact with the spinous processes of the lower cervical and upper thoracic spine.

Figure 16.24. Arms and hands d Once again the intention of this contact, as you can see now with my hands supporting the client, is to sense Primary Respiration between my two hands through her entire left arm and shoulder. This is also good work for the heart.

Figure 16.25. Atlas-occiput a (skeleton with labels) This image begins a sequence of work to come into relationship with the atlanto-occipital area. Here I am holding the occiput in my right hand and the atlas and axis in my left hand. This is an extremely important area of the body and of key interest in biodynamic craniosacral therapy.

Figure 16.26. Atlas-occiput b Here I have my hands in a similar position to the heart fulcrum, except the tips of my fingers are in the suboccipital triangle muscles. My ring and small fingers are in contact with the occiput. It is important to rest in this position in order to get a sense of any congestion in the area with the lymphatic system, tightness in the soft tissue, or irregular positioning of the atlas on the occiput.

Figure 16.27. Atlas-occiput c Here my hands have shifted and I have brought them together as if holding a bowl of water. I will be cradling the head in the palm of my hand and using the fingertips to palpate the suboccipital area while the pads of my fingers are in contact with the occiput.

Figure 16.28. Atlas-occiput d Here I have turned the client's head to the right to show you how I position my fingers to make contact with the whole atlanto-occipital area.

Figure 16.29. Atlas-occiput e (skeleton with labels) Now that the head is cradled in my hand, I begin to adjust my middle fingers to be the primary contact with the atlanto-occipital space.

Figure 16.30. Atlas-occiput f Now that the fingers are in place, I will sometimes slightly flex my fingertips to make a more snug connection with the atlanto-occipital space.

Figure 16.31. Atlas-occiput g This image shows my fingers flexed into the atlanto-occipital space. This is a gradual progression and not the starting point with the fingers flexed. I will only flex my fingers with a client in this position if there is a long history of cervical trauma, such as motor vehicle accidents. Even with such trauma, I will wait at least three sessions before I would even consider flexing my fingers. While I am flexing my fingers, I am subtly rotating the client's head with just a slight amount of micro movement to the right and left. Then I will also motion test with micro movement, sidebending her right ear to her right shoulder and her left ear to her left shoulder. The key is micro movement, not exceeding more than a quarter to a half an inch of movement in any direction. The motion is only used for several seconds followed by waiting and listening for several minutes for the autonomic nervous system to disengage. The head will get heavy, the soft tissue will relax, and the neck will lengthen.

Figure 16.32. Atlas-occiput h There are some times when a deeper level of the atlanto-occipital area needs to relax and disconnect from over use of the eyes, especially staring at computer screens. Here I asked the client to look to the left.

Figure 16.33. Atlas-occiput i Then I asked the client to look to the right while I moved the head very gently in the opposite direction. Again, I do not exceed more than a quarter to a half an inch of movement. It is easy to sense in which direction of eye gaze that the suboccipital area locks up or gets tighter. Then I ask the client to close the eyes and relax and I just wait for the upper cervical spine to soften. Again, this is a gradual series of skills with the atlanto-occipital area and the eye gazing skill is a skill of last resort in biodynamic practice.

Figure 16.34. Atlas-occiput-dural tube traction (skeleton) Here my hands are located in the region of the atlanto-occipital space. I am not lifting the cranium, but rather supporting the occiput and upper cervical spine. I like to visualize the entire dural tube filled with the spinal cord floating in cerebrospinal fluid from the foramen magnum down to the second sacral segment. I intend one microgram of cephalad (superior) traction on the client's occiput. I gradually sense my way down the dural tube as it softens. I hold some of my attention on Primary Respiration breathing the whole.

Figure 16.35. Heart tube a (skeleton) This image shows my hands making contact with the sternum on top and the upper thoracic spine below. The intention is to be able to sense the original embryonic tube. It is a fascial envelope that holds the lungs and heart in place.

Figure 16.36. Heart tube b Here I am with my hands on the client for sensing her heart tube. My body position is very important. Once again, my left elbow is supported by a pillow. In addition, if my head, which cannot be seen, is over or near the client's head, I need to turn my head so that when I exhale, she does not feel my breath on her face. This can be very distracting for a client.

Chapter 17: The Face

Figure 17.1. Mandible developmental movements This image shows the edge of my thumbs bilaterally on the client's mandible. I have contact with part of the masseter muscle as well as the lower border of the mandible. There are two developmental movements that the mandible makes after birth. Breastfeeding requires an anterior-posterior movement of the mandible and TMJ. Eating solid food requires a superior-inferior movement. Sensing Primary Respiration allows the mandible to self-correct in one or the other developmental movement.

Figure 17.2. Hyoid bone a (skeleton with labels) This image shows my fingers making bilateral contact with the hyoid bone. In actual practice, it is not necessary to make physical contact with it. Biodynamic practice is oriented around sensing the horizontal folds of the pharyngeal arches of the embryo. These horizontal folds breathe medially and laterally with Primary Respiration.

Figure 17.3. Hyoid bone b Here you can see my fingers near the client's hyoid bone. Please note the crease in her skin, which is a remnant of the pharyngeal arch. Since most people have this crease, it is an easy landmark to find.

Figure 17.4. Hyoid bone c This image shows my fingers as if they were holding a bowl of water near the hyoid bone. It is important to not make contact with the ears bilaterally. The palms are sensing the lateral fluctuations of the fluid body in the cranium. Again the orientation is to sense a lateral-medial movement at the rate of Primary Respiration.

Figure 17.5. Mandible a I want to demonstrate several different ways to make contact with the mandible. The mandible is the next pharyngeal arch above the hyoid. This image shows my index finger making contact on the lower border of the client's mandible bilaterally around the ramus.

Figure 17.6. Mandible b This image shows a bilateral contact with my middle fingers directly on the ramus of the mandible or on the inferior border of it.

Figure 17.7. Mandible c This hand position is a very comprehensive way to make contact with the lower border of the mandible as well as the masseter and temporalis muscles. It is important to remember that the contact must be very buoyant around the face whenever full-handed contact is used.

Figure 17.8. Temporomandibular joint a (skeleton with labels) I like to make a very simple bilateral contact with the tips of my middle fingers right over the joint space of the TMJ. Observe how my hands are positioned as if holding a bowl of water. The TMJ is a very sophisticated joint space and requires a comprehensive understanding and set of clinical skills. It is not possible for me to demonstrate such work in this book at this time.

Figure 17.9. Temporomandibular joint b This image shows the pads of my index and middle finger slightly below the TMJ on the bellies of the masseter muscles. This is intended to be a bilateral contact. Frequently the masseter carries a lot of tension and must soften for the TMJ to relax. Of course there are other deeper muscles associated with the TMJ. I am only going to show external work at this time. This means I will not be showing any intraoral work.

Figure 17.10. Maxilla a (skeleton with labels) Here I am making bilateral contact with the maxilla. Once again, my hands are positioned as if holding a bowl of water. The maxilla is the next pharyngeal arch above the mandible. The instructions are the same as the arches below it. I like to sense Primary Respiration breathing laterally and medially through the fluid fields of the face.

Figure 17.11. Maxilla b This image shows my fingers bilaterally on the client's maxilla. The superior landmark is the zygomatic bones. I let my fingers rest below the zygomatic bones and come into contact close to the upper teeth (externally). It is important that both arms be supported in order to stabilize the finger contact with any position on the face.

Figure 17.12. Transverse sinus There are several ways to make contact with the transverse sinus. Here the client's occiput is resting in the pads of my fingers. The pads of my fingers are located along the occipital border of the transverse sinus. The transverse sinus is a very important junction of the tentorium and vascular system of the cranium.

Figure 17.13. Anterior-posterior fluid fields a This is a hand position for the fluid fields of the face. My right hand is cupping the client's occiput and my middle finger is approximating the location of the transverse sinus. My left hand is making very light contact with the frontal bone. I like to sense Primary Respiration breathing between my two hands in the anterior-posterior dimension. Gradually, I wait for the fluid fields of the face to balance from front to back in the cranium.

Figure 17.14. Anterior-posterior fluid fields b (skeleton) My hands are positioned as before. This skull is a smaller than the client's head; consequently, my index finger is approximating the transverse sinus. I'm also using my top hand to palm the frontal bone. In this way, I am cradling the entire cranium. It is important to note that the practitioner's hands have to adapt and change to the size of the client's cranium. This is a very important fluid field to balance from anterior to posterior.

Figure 17.15. Ethmoid a There are many ways to make contact with the ethmoid bone. This image shows a thumb contact over the glabella of the frontal bone. The ethmoid bone is caudal to the frontal bone in this image. The rest of my hand is making a very light contact, and as the fluid fields of the face breathe laterally, the thumbs will depress as if the hands were like wings. When Primary Respiration changes direction, the reverse of that motion will occur. The ethmoid bone will lift the thumbs and the wings of the hands will settle down closer to the face.

Figure 17.16. Ethmoid b Many clients have had facial trauma. Occasionally, I mechanically attempt to loosen the ethmoid bone before balancing it biodynamically. My left hand is cupping the client's frontal bone. My right hand is making contact with the lacrimal bones. I then induce a very gentle torsion motion. My left hand rotates one direction while my right hand goes in the opposite with perhaps several ounces of pressure. I will do this for several seconds in each direction, and then I will stop and allow the face to breathe with Primary Respiration.

Figure 17.17. Ethmoid c Here my left hand is in the same position cupping the frontal bone. The thumb and index finger of my right hand are making contact with the client's maxilla. The instructions are the same as in the previous figure. This hand position is done in conjunction with the previous one in order to get a more thorough sense of freedom in the ethmoid bone without using intraoral work. It is important if using this type of skill to balance the fluid fields of the face with Primary Respiration.

Figure 17.18. Intraorbital ligament a (skeleton) This hand position combines a contact around the ethmoid with the pad of my left index finger and contact with the intraorbital ligament with the pad of my right index finger. The intraorbital ligament is responsible in prenatal development for pulling the eyes from the sides of the head into their normal anatomical position.

Figure 17.19. Intraorbital ligament b Here you can see my finger pads around the same position on the client's face. When synchronizing with Primary Respiration at this level, one finger moves down while the other is lifted up in rhythmic periods of fifty seconds. This is very relaxing for the eyes and the face in general.

Figure 17.20. Frontal bone This is a beautiful hand position where the index, middle, and ring fingers are making bilateral contact with the client's frontal bone. Originally, the frontal bone had a suture in the middle above the nose and, when the bone begins to breathe with Primary Respiration, it feels as if a bird is flying. The sides of the frontal bone lift up like wings and then go back down.

Figure 17.21. Full face This particular hand position is designed to sense the entire face responding to Primary Respiration. As with some of the previous facial hand positions, this hand position also gives a sense of a bird lifting off. Note that my thumbs are over the ethmoid bone. It is important to sense the movement of the ethmoid bone in relationship to all the facial bones. This hand position and many others for the face are very beneficial for balancing the parasympathetic nervous system.

Figure 17.22. Face in sidelying Occasionally, some clients are not able to lie in the supine position for very long. As you can see here, my hands are supporting the client's face. My right hand is below the ear and my left hand is above. Once again, I take time to sense Primary Respiration and allow the cranium to balance itself.

Chapter 18: The Cranial Vault and Base

Figure 18.1. Cranial preparatory window As I prepare to make contact with the client's cranial vault or cranial base, I always recommend having the hands lateral of the head, as you see here. I like to spend several minutes as if I'm holding a bowl of water. Then I like to sense Primary Respiration breathing the bowl of water into my hands and back from the center of the client's cranium.

Figure 18.2. Parietal lift a (skeleton with labels) I am making contact with the parietal bones at the inferior lateral angle (ILA). I like to use just the pad of my middle finger. The common name for this position is the parietal lift. Gradually, the movement of the parietal bones, much like that of the wings of a bird, becomes apparent. Then the motion of the superior leaf of the tentorium becomes apparent. I stay synchronized with Primary Respiration until the bones naturally float.

Figure 18.3. Parietal lift b Here you can see my finger contact by the inferior lateral angle of the parietal bones. As much as possible, my hands are extending and pretending to hold a bowl of water. I like to use this hand position when I am not sure where to begin on a client's cranium. Since there is no pressure on the parietal bones, it can be quite relaxing and decompressing for the client.

Figure 18.4. Parietal lift c This is the more traditional hand position for the parietal lift. The pads of my fingers are on the client's parietal ridge. Either hand position can be effective for sensing the motion of the parietal bones in relationship to the tentorium. It must be remembered that most of the cranial nerves traverse the space between the superior and inferior leafs of the tentorium.

Figure 18.5. Temporal lift a This image shows my hands stacked upon one another. My right hand is over my left hand. This is the starting hand position for coming into relationship with the mastoid process of the temporal bone.

Figure 18.6. Temporal lift b (skeleton with labels) Here you can see that the majority of the cranium is being supported in the palm of my right hand and only a little by the left hand. It is obvious that my thumb is posterior to the mastoid process of the temporal bone. The inferior leaf of the tentorium attaches to the petrous ridge of the temporal bone.

Figure 18.7. Temporal lift c Here my hands are in position cupping Valerie's head. It's important to make sure that the thumb is posterior to the mastoid process, as shown here. The temporal bones move in such a way that the mastoid process dips down and in medially at the same time, as if it were a wobbly wheel, and then reverses itself. Likewise the tentorium underneath the bones is moving in a lateral medial direction. It is important to sense the entire tentorium breathing and then the entire cranium breathing with Primary Respiration.

Figure 18.8. Temporal bones a (skeleton) This is a bilateral contact with my thumbs directly on the mastoid processes of the temporal bones.

Figure 18.9. Temporal bones b (skeleton with labels) In this view, I clearly show both of my thumbs in position over the mastoid processes.

Figure 18.10. Temporal bones c Here you can see my right hand in position on the client's temporal bone. My thumb fits snugly under the client's ear. The rest of my fingers simply rest wherever they land. The intention is clearly to sense the external and internal rotation of the temporal bones, both through the motion of the temporal squama and mastoid process.

Figure 18.11. Temporal bones d This view shows my hands in bilateral contact with the client's temporal bones. This is a great place to listen more directly to the fluid fields of the cranial base and how they breathe with Primary Respiration. Traditionally, it was taught that the temporal bones would stillpoint at the end of its phase of external rotation. From a biodynamic point of view, this may or may not happen, according to the intentions of Primary Respiration.

Figure 18.12. Traditional vault hold a This is the traditional vault hold to contact the cranial base via the greater wings of the sphenoid and the occiput.

In this image, you can see the pad of my left index finger over the greater wing of the sphenoid. My middle finger is very gently over the TMJ. My ring finger is in back of the ear along the temporal bone. My little finger, which is out of sight, is wedged very gently between the client's cranium and the table.

Figure 18.13. Traditional vault hold b This image shows the bilateral contact over the greater wings of the sphenoid. I shifted my body to the left, as you can see by the position of my wrists, for the photographer to take this image.

Figure 18.14. Traditional vault hold c Here I have rotated the client's head to the left to show the full hand contact on the right side of the client's cranium. My little finger is in clear view on the occiput and the palm of my hand is over the parietal bones. My thumb is in contact with the frontal bone. Please remember that thumbs have a tendency to flex and compress the client's cranium. With this traditional vault hold, the practitioner must have a sensory awareness not only of the location, but the depth of contact that every square millimeter of the hand is making with the client's head.

Figure 18.15. Traditional vault hold d This is a lateral view of my right hand resting in its position for the vault hold. The vault hold is used biodynamically to sense the metabolic fields that formed the cranial base in utero. It is essential to sense Primary Respiration breathing the cranial base. In addition, some practitioners place a foot extender on the treatment table in order to have more of the forearm parallel with the client's body.

Figure 18.16. Sphenoid decompression This is a hand position I sometimes use with clients who have had facial trauma. I am exclusively monitoring the movement of the greater wings of the sphenoid with the pads of my thumbs. Sometimes, the sphenoid does need to be mechanically decompressed because of trauma. The action is to very gently, with micrograms of pressure, traction the sphenoid up toward the ceiling. This is only done for several seconds at a time. Then the practitioner must pause and let the cranial base breathe with Primary Respiration.

Figure 18.17. Becker hold a (skeleton with labels) This hand position is an alternative way to approach the cranial base. This image simply shows the relationship of the basiocciput with the basisphenoid. The only thing missing here to fill out the cranial base is the petrous ridge of the temporal bones.

Figure 18.18. Becker hold b (skeleton with labels) Here you can see the edge of my thumbs over the greater wing of the sphenoid and the edge of my middle finger, ring finger, and little finger gently wedged between the cranium and the table and thus in contact with the occiput.

Figure 18.19. Becker hold c Here are my hands on the client's cranial base via the greater wing of the sphenoid and the occiput. This is a much easier way to come into relationship with the metabolic fields that form the cranial base. I am also able to shape my hands as if holding a bowl of water. Remember that Primary Respiration is the key to sensing the normalization of the cranial base.

Figure 18.20. Becker hold d Here Valerie's hands are on my head. Valerie's hands are smaller than mine. It is important that if a practitioner has smaller hands, the main contact with the cranial base comes through the occiput. Valerie's thumb is resting slightly below the greater wing of my sphenoid. Nonetheless the motion of the metabolic fields is still available.

Figure 18.21. Occiput CV4 a (skeleton with labels) Traditionally, CV4 means compression of the fourth ventricle. The practitioner, however, is offering very subtle compression when appropriate. In order to support the squamous portion of the occiput on the thenar eminences of the thumbs, the hands need to be positioned as shown. Notice my thenar eminences because of their thickness. This is where the occiput needs to rest and sometimes I need to rotate my thumbs out a little bit so the client's head can find the sweet, soft spot at the base of my thumbs.

Figure 18.22. Occiput CV4 b Now my hands are in position just medial of the occipitomastoid suture. Some authorities claim that the occiput is the primary stress bone in the birth process. Consequently, the occipital-mastoid suture may be fixated in such a way that the fourth ventricle does not have a full range of motion available to it.

Figure 18.23. Occiput CV4 c Here my hands are supporting the client's occiput. The occiput has its greatest range of motion by the occipital mastoid suture. Consequently, I begin to sense the lateral-medial motion of the bone and wait until the entire cranium begins to slow down and has an opportunity to choose whether it wants to take a pause, which is traditionally called a still-point.

Figure 18.24. The bird in the ventricles This is an image by a student and assistant of mine in Germany, Josefine Frind. She drew it some years ago for her class project in one of my classes. The outline of the ventricles can be seen almost like a watermark in the middle of the bird. It is this sensibility that the practitioner is attempting to palpate.

Figure 18.25. Igniting the bird a (skeleton) I want to begin showing a sequence to come into relationship with the third ventricle. The contact with my right hand is once again with the index finger over the greater wing of the sphenoid. My thumbs are crossed and gently making contact with bregma. Please note that my wrists and arms need to be properly supported, which they are not in this photo. I forgot to roll up a towel and place it under my wrists. Next time I will remember to do this.

Figure 18.26. Igniting the bird b Here you can see my arms properly supported on the table. My thumbs are crossed in a way that the pad of my right thumb has contact with bregma and the pads of my index fingers have contact with the greater wings of the sphenoid. I sometimes call this palpation "the bird in the ventricle." As the thumbs begin to sense the midline of the ventricles in their rhythmic motion with Primary Respiration, the greater wings of the sphenoid will open and close like the wings of a bird.

Figure 18.27. Igniting the bird c Here you can see my hands on Valerie's head. The contacts are the same as above. I want to be able to feel the flight of the bird in the ventricles. The third ventricle is the heart of the bird. The fourth ventricle is the tail of the bird. The lateral ventricles, neural tissue, and greater wings of the sphenoid bone represent the wings of the bird. Let the ventricles fly with Primary Respiration.

Chapter 19: Anterior Midline

Figure 19.1. Anterior midline a (skeleton) The anterior midline is an embryological seam from bregma to the pubic symphysis. It represents the last phase of closure over the ventral surface of the body, which does not take place until several months after birth. The first position is a finger contact on bregma and the intraorbital ligament sensing Primary Respiration.

Figure 19.2. Anterior midline b Here my finger placement for the first position on the client's head can be seen. Sometimes I go through this process while I am seated to the side of the client and other times I will do it standing. It does not make a lot of difference, except that in both cases, the arms need to have stable support.

Figure 19.3. Anterior midline c (skeleton) In the next position, I merely overlap my fingers such that one finger remains on the intraorbital ligament and the other makes contact with the philtrum, the medial groove of the upper lip.

Figure 19.4. Anterior midline d Here you can see my finger placement on the client's face with the intraorbital ligament and philtrum. Once again the focus is on sensing Primary Respiration in any dimension.

Figure 19.5. Anterior midline e (skeleton) Here I have switched my fingers so that one remains on the philtrum and the other is on the mentalis of the mandible. The mentalis was originally a suture dividing the mandible into two portions.

Figure 19.6. Anterior midline f Here you can see my finger placement on the client's face over the philtrum and mentalis. I focus on Primary Respiration.

Figure 19.7. Anterior midline g (skeleton) The next position involves a finger contact remaining on the mentalis and the other finger on the sternoclavicular notch.

Figure 19.8. Anterior midline h Here is that same finger placement on the client's face and upper sternum. My fingers are making contact with the mentalis and sternoclavicular notch. I am using my index fingers exclusively to sense Primary Respiration.

Figure 19.9. Anterior midline i (skeleton) This image shows one finger remaining on the sternoclavicular notch and the other finger on the xyphoid process at the bottom of the sternum.

Figure 19.10. Anterior midline j Now my hands are on the trunk of the client's body. I am using my middle finger for contact with the sternoclavicular notch and xyphoid process. Here my hands are over the heart and pericardium and Primary Respiration can be sensed more directly in and around the heart and respiratory diaphragm.

Figure 19.11. Anterior midline k (skeleton) The next position involves one contact remaining on the xyphoid process and the other finger over the umbilicus. One has to imagine that since this is a skeleton, the index finger of my left hand is approximating the location of the umbilicus.

Figure 19.12. Anterior midline l Here are my hands with the placement over the xyphoid and umbilicus. For the sake of the reader being able to see the umbilicus, I have moved my middle finger of my right hand slightly lateral of the umbilicus. Normally, the finger would be over the umbilicus.

Figure 19.13. Anterior midline m (skeleton) In this image, one finger is remaining over the umbilicus and the other finger in contact with the pubic symphysis. This is the last hand position for the anterior midline.

Figure 19.14. Anterior midline n Here is the final hand placement over the client's anterior midline. If the practitioner does not know where the pubic symphysis is located in the client, the client can be asked to show where it is located. All of these hand positions involve sensing Primary Respiration. I am frequently asked if the entire sequence needs to be done each time the anterior midline is approached. The answer is no, but it is important to practice all of them periodically in order to differentiate when it is appropriate to use all or some of the hand positions for the anterior midline.

CHAPTER 21

Biodynamic Therapeutic Processes

Client palpation is the phase in a cycle of attunement when the practitioner places attention on his or her own hands at the surface of the client's skin. This is called a window of observation. The practitioner is taking the pulse of the client's fluid body much like an acupuncturist checks a client's meridian pulses at the beginning and end of an acupuncture session. The quality of the client's fluid body pulse frequently determines the biodynamic therapeutic process that will unfold or be facilitated by the practitioner. What is the pulse of the fluid body? Is it able to expand and contract or breathe three dimensionally at the rate of Primary Respiration? This capacity describes the first and perhaps most important biodynamic therapeutic process.

In this chapter I will describe three principal biodynamic therapeutic processes. First is the client's whole three-dimensional fluid body breathing with Primary Respiration. I feel that this is the most important biodynamic therapeutic process. How does a practitioner help to ignite the client's fluid body or improve its pulse? If the fluid body has a weak pulse, then the second biodynamic therapeutic process becomes the focus of a session: helping to establish a stable autonomic nervous system in the client. Such stabilization invites the possibility of a neutral or starting point for a biodynamic therapeutic process in which the autonomic nervous systems of the practitioner and client disengage from high or low tone states and Primary Respiration is free to enhance its reparation of the fluid body. This is described in detail in Chapters 5 through 9. Once the fluid body starts to breathe properly and the autonomics are stable, the midline of the client may manifest.

The third biodynamic therapeutic process is reconnecting the client to the natural world through zone practice. Attention is directed to other aspects of the therapeutic process unfolding in and around the client, especially the natural world. Zone practice, detailed in Chapter 5, is based on the practitioner performing a cycle of attunement regularly in a session. Since zone practice is a perceptual skill performed before and during contact with the client, I will not focus on that in this chapter. I have covered it thoroughly in previous chapters.

237

The transition from localized motion present in the client's anatomy and physiology to the breathing of the whole fluid body via Primary Respiration is frequently missed by inexperienced practitioners. Thus the purpose of this final chapter is to help organize the practitioner's use of the windows described with all the photographs in the preceding chapters. I would also like to state two principles again:

- The biodynamic therapeutic process is initiated by the quality of the practitioner's attention first in his or her own body and then through the zones that include the client.

- The practitioner must self-ignite his or her own fluid body first, which generates a resonance with the client's nervous system and heart. The client must be able to orient to the practitioner's nervous system and heart. This opens the door to the breathing biodynamic therapeutic process.

Varieties of Therapeutic Processes

The practitioner's hands are frequently placed in specific locations on the client's body relating to developmental anatomy. The embryology must be known from accurate images of the embryo and visualized in the practitioner's body and occasionally around the client's body. These so-called embryological windows are windows to observe the biodynamic therapeutic process governed by Primary Respiration and its interchange with the Dynamic Stillness. When the window of observation allows the embryo to emerge as a breathing whole in the relationship between practitioner and client, it is a biodynamic therapeutic process. The embryo and its movements are an access point to a biodynamic embryonic process under the direction of Primary Respiration. There are, of course, descriptions of therapeutic processes in the Mid Tide level of work taught, such as the inherent treatment plan employed by many schools. I am not talking about that level of work, which is quite valid. Traditional craniosacral therapy mentions such processes as the state of balanced membrane tension, which is related but not the subject of this or any of my books. At the most mechanical level, the therapeutic process is completely dictated by the practitioner. I remember being told many years ago by an osteopath, "Find it, fix it, leave it alone."

Many of the photographs in this book are based on discovering the embryo in the client. The ground of observation, however, is not limited to the practitioner's hands but rather his or her entire body. The key point with the embryology is to sense and visualize wholeness in one's own body. Wholeness is the smallest subdivision of life. The hands and arms are simply like an umbilical cord connecting aspects of the whole such as the embryo and placenta. Much of Volume Three demonstrated that principle.

What follows here is a description of the three biodynamic therapeutic processes of establishing living, breathing wholeness as the ground of healing, stabilizing the autonomic nervous system of the client, and finally reconnecting the client to the natural world with palpation and perceptual skills. Think of these three explorations as the *principal biodynamic therapeutic processes.* There are likely many related processes yet to be uncovered.

A biodynamic session is rarely a linear process as described here or in the many photographs in this book. One or none of these biodynamic therapeutic processes may be available in any given session. Perhaps a therapeutic session is simply about waiting in peace. The practitioner must be ready to deal with the frustration of nothing happening with the client and avoid provoking a response when feeling bored or frustrated. But when one of the three biodynamic therapeutic processes occurs, the practitioner observes that process with the client while synchronized with Primary Respiration and stillness.

Wholeness

All windows seek to establish a container of wholeness and three-dimensional symmetry in both the practitioner's and client's body. This is a suggested starting point that in application may unfold in a very nonlinear way. I have had some clients come in with a lot of physical pain and sometimes I simply put my hands on where it hurts to begin a session. Relating to specific symptoms in the client's body, however, usually comes later if it is necessary at all. I resist approaching the location of the client's symptoms for three sessions to see if the wholeness of Primary Respiration is helpful. It usually is.

This is not a *fix-it* model, although symptom reduction frequently does occur in the client and must be respected as one of any number of possibilities in the client's healing process that I described in Volume Three. The Pietà window is used most frequently to establish this sensibility and to take the pulse of the client's fluid body. Holding the feet bilaterally, the shoulders bilaterally, and the sacrum are also excellent for establishing this intention, especially if the practitioner is sitting in one position for prolonged periods of time.

Fluid Body

The primary biodynamic therapeutic process is to be able to ignite the fluid body and reestablish its breathing function with Primary Respiration. Any window will support this intention, but specifically the fulcrum of the fluid body around the respiratory diaphragm is particularly valuable because of the relationship of Primary and secondary respiration. The windows for the umbilicus are also excellent because of gut issues, as discussed in the first four chapters of this volume. Finally, the window for the sacrum and primitive streak allows a much deeper rehabilitation of the fluid body, because of the relationship of the pelvic floor and pelvic-floor issues from the past that influence the fluid body. This was discussed in Chapter 15 regarding the longitudinal fluctuation at the coccyx and further on in this chapter.

Occasionally, a phase of the biodynamic therapeutic process within the fluid body will be initiated by a sense of idling or stillness in the fluid body. This is a function of buoyancy. Thus it is important for the practitioner to orient to his or her own sense of three-dimensional buoyancy and sense of lift in his or her whole fluid body to create a resonance for the client. Igniting the fluid body will generate autonomic stability. This is sometimes called a neutral or wholistic shift. It is most frequently accompanied by a sense of Dynamic Stillness occurring in and around the client in any of the zones and a sense of buoyancy in the practitioner's fluid body. This is a valuable biodynamic therapeutic process that leads to the joy of sensing three-dimensional buoyancy. I am associating the felt sense of joy with this biodynamic therapeutic process.

This is one of the reasons all of the windows require different types of perception, awareness, and mindfulness that I define in the Glossary, which follows this chapter. Perception includes zone phenomena, Primary Respiration interchanging with stillness, and other rates specific to the function of the fluid body such as the Mid Tide. Before a neutral occurs, contact with the client is an exploration of wholeness and stability in the autonomic nervous system, as I will discuss below. After the neutral, the same windows support the further ignition of the fluid body and eventually the restoration of its functional midline and ultimately a reconnection with nature.

Heat

The next level of support for the fluid body to breath as a whole is to build the fire (heat) in the blood and heart. Primary Respiration has a direct relationship with the heat in the body. The fire builds the wind and the wind of Primary Respiration builds the fire. This reciprocal elemental relationship between these two aspects of biology generates the potency or life force. These in turn generate the fluid body and the remaining earthy elements of the body such as the autonomic nervous system. This relationship can be evoked from any of the above explorations, especially regarding the autonomic nervous system. The thermoregulatory system of the body, both neurologically and cardiovascularly, is all about the heat necessary to create, repair, and maintain the life of the fluid body. It is the release and permeation of heat we feel in our own body and the client's during a session that is really a vitally important part of the biodynamic therapeutic process. Specific windows such as the bilateral SBJ (sphenobasilar junction) window can influence the hypothalamus where the thermoregulatory center of the brain is located. Windows related to the heart and attention on the blood are also incredibly valuable as the heart warms the blood and distributes warmth through the body.

The heat I refer to here requires the practitioner to pay attention to his or her breathing patterns and to notice when he or she takes a spontaneous deep breath. I advise students to take three to five deep breaths during every session in order to synchronize Primary and secondary respiration. Dr. Sutherland was fond of getting his clients to do deep breathing at critical points in the therapeutic process such as the beginning of Primary Respiration expansion. In general, if a practitioner is going to verbally solicit a deep breath from the client, it is synchronized with the phase of Primary Respiration as it is beginning to expand. Thus the breath in its ignition function is an important adjunct to the biodynamic therapeutic process related to establishing the permeation of heat in the fluid body and soma. The practitioner is responsible for self-igniting this therapeutic heat system. This means spending time synchronizing Primary and secondary respiration during a session. The practitioner orients to buoyancy first, then synchronizes Primary and secondary respiration in himself or herself.

Stabilizing the Autonomic Nervous System

Almost all windows can be used to observe a biodynamic therapeutic process with the autonomic nervous system. It is always attempting to stabilize itself. When the pulse of the fluid body is weak or not available, the biodynamic therapeutic process for helping the client is to self-regulate one's autonomic nervous system in order to reduce fear and increase the felt sense of safety in the client. In general, when the quality of contact is extremely gentle and buoyant, coupled with regular cycles of attunement in the zones, this lends itself to self-regulation of the autonomic nervous system in the practitioner and the client. It is really the ground of biodynamic practice. Holding the extremities, especially the feet, is excellent for disengaging high and low tone in the autonomic nervous system. Holding a client's hand, one side at a time, is also an excellent way to begin reducing fear, which is regulated by the amygdala in the temporal lobes of the brain. Whenever holding a client's hand, the practitioner must verbally solicit the client's comfort level. Certain forms of trauma immobilize the arms and hands and holding them may be contraindicated.

Palpation can be applied with variable degrees of depth and pressure. This depends on the training a practitioner has undertaken and his or her instinct for nonintrusive depth and pressure, which is a function of experience. The embryo and adult share an outer layer of tissue and an inner limiting tissue. The inner limiting tissue under the skin in the adult is where the watery element of the embryo begins. If the practitioner is using more pressure, attention is diffused through that watery element at any depth of palpation by sensing from the backs of the practitioner's hands, as detailed in Chapter 10. Regardless of the depth and pressure, the practitioner always needs to keep his or her eyes open for signs of activation in the autonomic nervous system of the client. This is covered in detail in Volume Two.

In general, contact with the surface of the client's skin through the clothes begins with a very light touch and is verbally negotiated with the client for comfort level regarding depth and pressure. What the practitioner considers as appropriate pressure may be quite different from the client's experience of the same touch. The practitioner needs to verbally solicit the client's comfort level periodically if it appears that the client is awake, fidgeting, or keeping the eyes open. Finally, at an advanced level, the autonomic nervous system of the client is best contacted through the zone B of the practitioner meeting zone B of the client, as discussed in Chapter 5 and shown in Figure 5.3.

The Diaphragms

A structural orientation to stabilizing the client's autonomic nervous system is done through the diaphragms as a whole. They are the pelvic, respiratory, thoracic, atlanto-occipital space, diaphragm of sellae, and tentorium cerebelli diaphragms. Some authors include the feet and knees as diaphragms. There are many windows for making contact with the diaphragms of the body; I have included several in Chapters 15 and 16. These windows generally support regulation of the autonomic nervous system as the diaphragms are densely innervated by the autonomic nervous system. In addition, the diaphragms are considered to be space organizers for the fascial system of the body in the sense of being like scaffolding around which the three-dimensional structure of the body is formed. Needless to say, the diaphragms are important at many levels structurally and functionally in establishing the shape and function of wholeness in the body. The breathing function of the respiratory diaphragm is considered to be the oldest function in our fluid body. All diaphragms breathe in unison with the respiratory diaphragm. This breathing is linked to Primary Respiration. It is vitally important that the breathing of the diaphragms be synchronized with Primary Respiration.

The Heart

Another set of windows is used to balance the cardiovascular system because of its influence on helping to regulate the autonomic nervous system at the level of the hypothalamus in the brain. These windows are located anywhere around the rib cage and spine, either anterior around the sternum and clavicles or posterior on the spine, scapulae, and rib cage. This would also include windows related to the liver, the heart, the lungs, and intestines, all shown in Chapter 15. In addition, the window for balancing the heart fulcrum at C3 (third cervical vertebra) is particularly valuable in establishing such balance. If a client has either a hyposensitive or hypersensitive autonomic nervous system, the practitioner needs to focus attention on the cardiovascular system. Again this is done with the practitioner's hands attending to the inner limiting tissue and the watery element that is embedded in the blood capillaries. The biodynamic therapeutic process in this case is through the attention on the three-dimensional nature of the blood and heart. The capillaries have a distinct sensibility and are worthy of the practitioner's exploration because they are just beneath the surface of the skin.

The Cranium

The cranium has a direct relationship to stability in the autonomic nervous system. This is because each of the three sections of the cranium are formed from different metabolic fields in the embryo. Each part of the cranium behaves a bit differently locally within the whole breathing fluid body of the cranium because of the individual metabolic fields associated with the cranium in general. There really are no distinct tissue boundaries between these three sections of the cranium from a biodynamic embryological point of view. Any windows on the cranium, including those on the face, the vault, and the base shown in this book, are directly influencing the autonomic nervous system. Contact, especially on the vault and the base, is not generally used in the early stages of biodynamic treatment. It is premature to do so in biodynamic practice. The face however, may be contacted as early as possible in a series of treatments. It is the genetic mediator of growth for the brain and heart developmentally. Think of the face as between the heart and brain and then imagine allowing it to decompress. This directly influences the heart and brain. The face is also an extension of the upper end of the gastrointestinal system and thus considered to be a core-level structure.

Working with the face in a series of treatments must be done cautiously. But it will produce one of the largest veins of gold, in terms of being able to support the biodynamic therapeutic processes of returning to wholeness and stabilizing the autonomic nervous system. One teacher has said that there is a lot of "heavy traffic" in the head whether from birth process, dental trauma, concussions, multitasking visually, or physical abuse. Great caution must be used when working with any aspect of the cranium, which is why I do not teach contacting the cranium until my fourth or fifth level of the basic training. This is because the therapeutic relationship is a two-person biology; the client's cranium can actually reflect the practitioner's birth patterns. The clinical progression I recommend is to wait until the second or third session in a series with a client and then contact the face first, followed by the vault and finally the base. Not all three (face, vault, and base) are generally contacted in one session. For example, if the face holds a lot of trauma that has been divulged to me on my intake form and client interview, then I will start with the cranial vault and usually the parietal lift as the most benign entry point in the cranium.

The other clinical value of working around the cranium in general and the face specifically has to do with repairing the autonomic nervous system and its social function (Porges, 2011). The face is related to what Stephen Porges calls the social nervous system. Thus another way of restoring healthy function in the social aspect (safety and trust) of the autonomic nervous system is to relate with the face. Human relationships require face-to-face contact for empathy and compassion to be a shared experience. Learning the relationship to the biodynamic therapeutic process through the face is achieved with contact via the metabolic fields of the fluid body, as detailed in previous volumes, and a description of the fields can be found in the Glossary. Contact with the fields is done via Primary Respiration in that whole area and waiting for one or the other of the fields to manifest in the practitioner's hands. Furthermore, the development of the face involves a horizontal movement based on the embryology of the face and an anterior-to-posterior movement. These movements in sum reflect the cranium as a breathing whole that must be related to the whole fluid body, and this depends on the global view of the client's body held by the practitioner. The biggest challenge I have consistently found on working with any aspect of the cranium is that it is compressive in nature because that is its developmental nature through the metabolic fields, and thus compression must be normalized through the perception of Primary Respiration and then related to the whole as mentioned.

Misattuned touch can trigger pre- and perinatal imprinting when attention to Primary Respiration via the cycle of attunement is lacking in the practitioner. This means normal feelings of compression in the client may become nonnormal and cascade into overactivation of the autonomic nervous system. This is what I call combustion in Chapter 9. In addition, the involuntary movements of the cranial bones, the meninges, and the neural tissue often appear in any or all windows on the cranium. These are Mid Tide movements or sometimes even faster tempos. I simply allow Primary Respiration, however, to become the focus of any fast or medium tempo that I encounter, except for the longitudinal fluctuation mentioned below. Windows for the cranium include bilateral contact with the sphenoid bone, temporal bones, parietal bones, and any position on the occiput. Any movement in the layers of the bones, meninges, and neural tissue must be joined to Primary Respiration and its interchange with stillness and then brought into relationship with the whole fluid body through the zones, as stated regularly throughout this book. All these layers must be balanced into one functioning whole without boundaries or layers. This is done through the fluid body. Consequently, the biodynamic therapeutic process of wholeness is the way to begin and end a session. The middle part of a session is the time to explore more local fluid body phenomena and tissue layering such as in the cranium.

The Midline

The next way of stabilizing the autonomic nervous system is to ignite the midline for the repair and restoration of its ordering structural and functional capacities. There are many structural midlines and that can be a problem with some biodynamic approaches. This is because a practitioner, thinking that igniting a structural midline is the goal of practice, prematurely compresses the client's midline, which can be retraumatizing (Levine, 2010). I feel that it is important to focus on the deepest functional aspect of the midline first and that means a Dynamic Stillness that is nonlocal. In other words, stillness as an expression of the midline may actually occur in any of the zones, especially zone C.

Stillness is the core of any midline from the notochord to the self-regulation capacity of the prefrontal cortex and the spiritual as well. The midline is all about stillness. It is vitally important to expand our definition of a midline as being capable of moving or automatically shifting from inside the client's body to outside and then back. In biodynamic practice, the focus is on establishing wholeness first with Primary Respiration, autonomic stability second, and so forth. A structural midline such as the notochord will naturally arise in its own time in the client. It cannot be forced or pushed because it is heavily defended in the contemporary client. The deeper experience of stillness will usually precede the localized manifestation of a structural midline.

The client is grounding him- or herself through the nervous system of the practitioner. This is the direction of flow that begins and ends a session. It necessarily includes the practitioner's movement of attention through the zones. Gradually the notochordal midline (structural) of the embryo or other organizational midlines will reveal themselves or not, in the practitioner's perception. The notochordal midline in the spine and basicranium is fundamentally related and responsive to the interchange of Primary Respiration (the metabolic fields that form the notochord) and stillness at its deepest level. Finally, it must be considered that this functional aspect of the midline of the client moves out and back through the zones, as I said above. Overemphasis on the midline is premature before establishing a breathing whole. In addition, the midline is a very personal thing spiritually, as I discussed in Volume One of this series. From a spiritual point of view, a practitioner cannot know the experience of the client's midline. Leave it alone, focus on the whole, and orient to stillness whenever possible and for as long as possible.

Practitioners must stop focusing on finding a midline in the client's body until it reveals itself either in the body or, most likely, outside the body. This is the biodynamic meaning of automatic shifting. I spent many years working with clients who had been in car accidents. Over time I realized how the client's nervous system had been displaced outside the body. By allowing the client to orient to the practitioner's nervous system and moving attention through the zones, the client's nervous system can reorient to its natural fulcrum and thus reestablish its natural ability to automatically shift. I believe this is the case with most trauma in general and the beauty of biodynamic work specifically.

Longitudinal Fluctuation

A very important organizational movement of the fluid body is the longitudinal fluctuation (LF) of the fluid body, from the coccyx up to the third ventricle. This has a very specific rate of two-and-a-half cycles per minute (2.5 CPM). It is a Mid Tide movement. The practitioner has to be led to this rate through Primary Respiration and not look for it directly, since it is frequently not available because of imprinting on the fluid body from drug usage, sexual abuse, and metabolic problems such as constipation related to diet. Please review the first four chapters in this volume to get a sense of how improper diet contributes to altered fluid body dynamics. The LF, as mentioned in Chapter 15, is the dynamic midline of the fluid body, which Sutherland described as the "direct current." It is this functional midline that is most frequently unavailable in the contemporary client, having been extinguished or greatly diminished by the combustion of traumatic stress and resulting speed generated by the autonomic nervous system. This refers to the function of hyperarousal/fight-flight and hypoarousal/freeze states in the autonomic nervous system. It results in too much heat being generated in the body and the metabolic response of encapsulating the heat within the area of trauma, which alters the flow through the body. An inability to thermally regulate is one of the hallmarks of traumatic stress and trauma in general. It also refers to claustrophobic thinking and racing thoughts common in people who experience traumatic stress or live with the effects of it every day. When a client has a side effect from a session with Primary Respiration, it may just be that the client's autonomic nervous system is overreacting to the stimulus of the touch. This again is a hallmark of people who have experienced trauma.

Obviously, direct and indirect palpation of the coccyx is necessary to sense the LF. It must be remembered that the practitioner must access his or her own pelvic floor and initiate a longitudinal fluctuation in his or her fluid body by using mild chi kung (qi gong) exercises, for example, that involve tightening the muscles of the pelvic floor in conjunction with conscious breathing to self-ignite the LF. This is detailed in Chapter 15.

I also will visualize the cycle of the LF going up to the third ventricle and cascading out around my zone B and recoalescing at my coccyx. I only do this briefly to see if the LF of the client can be ignited through the resonance of my LF. Because of sexual abuse and trauma, it is more important to establish a breathing wholeness with Primary Respiration in the fluid body of the client rather than prematurely igniting the longitudinal fluctuation. I mentioned earlier that working zone B to zone B between client and practitioner is an advanced practice for recalibrating the client's autonomic nervous system but also for sensing the return flow of the LF in zone B.

The LF, if it is not missing, can be heavily fortified and trigger strong reactions and side effects, such as headaches, nausea, depression, or anxiety, when it is approached prematurely by a practitioner or subtly compressed. This is why it is very important to take the pulse of the fluid body at the beginning and end of a session so the practitioner knows if it is getting stronger or not when certain windows and explorations are used. This is especially true for the LF. Take the pulse of the fluid body, check the availability of the LF, and then recheck the pulse of the whole fluid body. Recall that the LF is a pulse itself and it is associated with other pulses in the fulcrums of the fluid body that I mentioned in Chapter

15. Windows for either the notochordal midline or longitudinal fluctuation are going to be the coccyx, sacrum, spine, occiput, and sphenoid. In addition, the ethmoid bone and vomer bone are considered midline structures by osteopathic definition. But the attention of the practitioner is not in the client's midline but rather the hands are an offering, an invitation, for the midline to emerge in communion with the practitioner's attention to the whole at the surface of the client's fluid body.

Stillpoint

Stillpoint technology has been a part of the cranial concept from its earliest beginnings. The terms or acronyms CV4 (compression of the fourth ventricle) and EV4 (expansion of the fourth ventricle) traditionally describe windows located on the occiput and temporal bones, respectively. These traditional palpation skills biomechanically involve using compressive force on the occiput as an attempt to stop the movement of the cerebrospinal fluid (CSF) when the ventricles are at an end point of contraction in the normal movement cycle (CV4) or on the temporal bones at an end point of the normal phase of expansion (EV4). The normal movement cycles of the CSF are associated with fast and Mid Tide tempos. Temporary and purposeful stopping of this motion is said to rebalance the central nervous system and consequently the whole body. These are techniques of last resort and, yes, I still use them perhaps a couple of times a year—in less than one percent of my clients.

That same terminology, however, is used differently in biodynamic practice. A CV4 refers to the ability of the *whole fluid body* to temporarily become still at the end point of its contraction phase and just before expansion. The EV4 would simply be the reverse, in which there is a temporary stillness at the end point of expansion just before the contraction phase. Some osteopaths refer to a different tempo than the ones I have mentioned. There is a tempo between Primary Respiration and the longitudinal fluctuation; it is called the reciprocal tension potency (RTP) and has one cycle per minute—thirty seconds of contraction and thirty seconds of expansion. This is the tempo that biodynamic practitioners are working with for a biodynamic CV4 or EV4. The window at the scapulae is particularly valuable for sensing this capacity in the fluid body. Most any other window below the head of the client, especially the Pietà, could facilitate this perception. When the practitioner synchronizes his or her attention with this RTP tempo, it augments the therapeutic effect in the client. Frequently such a stillpoint is associated with establishing a neutral in the client and thus could ignite a biodynamic therapeutic process. As a rule of thumb in biodynamic practice, focus on EV4s rather than CV4s because a CV4 may compress the midline too much. A biodynamic, rather than a mechanical, CV4 allows Primary Respiration to expand three dimensionally and this is what the contemporary client needs most.

In conclusion, some windows are specifically used to enhance or ignite the therapeutic relationship. This is an important distinction in biodynamic practice as I teach and practice with my clients. This includes any window that employs a visualization of the embryo-uterine, fetal-uterine, or mother-infant relationship. Chapter 5 on the zones shows this in detail. Specific windows around the umbilicus are important biodynamic therapeutic processes for reconnecting the client with the natural world via zone practice. This is the biodynamic therapeutic process of establishing the relationship as a circulatory system or an interpersonal cardiovascular system. Volume Three focused on the therapeutic relationship involving the heart and cardiovascular system of both practitioner and client. Now, that metaphor must be extended out to zone D, the natural world. It is now well established that contact with nature is restorative to one's health and well-being (Barton and Pretty, 2010). Barton and Pretty established a link between having attention on nature and compassion. Thus it is through this biodynamic therapeutic relationship with client, self, and nature that a deeper level of empathy and compassion is established. This then leads to the emergence of altruistic love and kindness as the ultimate biodynamic therapeutic process. Biodynamic craniosacral therapy is thus a model of empathy and compassion.

I want to thank Tim Shafer and Marcel Bryner for their careful and thoughtful review of this chapter. Their editing has made it better for students and practitioners.

Seven Levels of Motion in the Cranium

Palpation of the cranium is based on being able to differentiate at least seven different levels of involuntary motion. There are several prerequisites. The first is working with the biodynamic process called attunement and the periodic perception of Primary Respiration in the practitioner. Then the practitioner maintains awareness of the back of the arms and hands, the head, the spine, and in general the whole posterior surface of his or her body. The practitioner needs to cultivate afferent hands that only sense the client and are free from motor activity and intention. Finally, the practitioner must also be able to clearly sense his or her own zone B first and then that of the client. These degrees of practitioner sensitivity and self-awareness are necessary since most clients have experienced impact trauma to the head at some point in their life.

The practitioner starts with his or her afferent hands lateral of the client's head by about six inches on either side. This is to tune into zone B of the client and synchronize with Primary Respiration out to the horizon and back. Then the practitioner places her or his hands on the skin or scalp of the client with equal attention to zone B of the client. At this interface, the practitioner waits for the movements and shapes of the cranium to come out to the surface or into zone B, which typically is above the skin out to about twenty inches. This is also called the "biosphere" by Dr. Becker or zone B by contemporary biodynamic cranial osteopaths. This perception means that the practitioner places more attention on the backs of his or her hands, rather than the palms and finger pads in order to maintain contact with zone B. Bearing all this in mind, here are seven levels of cranial motions from outside to inside with an understanding that in clinical practice these motions may appear randomly and rarely in this sequence:

- **Primary Respiration.** A 100-second cycle and related ignition events, either breathing the soma (zone A) of the practitioner or moving from the horizon (zone D) to the inside of the practitioner's body and back. Primary Respiration must be established as a perceptual reality in and around the practitioner first and then the client, especially when sensing the client's cranium. Furthermore, Primary Respiration gives the practitioner access to the metabolic fields of the body. The metabolic fields are still present in the adult body as active shaping processes underlying all structure and function.

- **The fluid body.** The fluid body is a single three-dimensional drop of viscous fluid living in the container of both zone A and zone B together. At the cranium, fluid movements typically move lateral to medial and inferior to anterior around a shifting fulcrum located in and around the third ventricle. If a practitioner focuses on the cranium alone, however, it can compress the client and create side effects. This is why the practitioner, when working around the cranium, must periodically envision the whole three-dimensional soma and fluid body of the client (zones A and B together). This includes practicing regular cycles of attunement out to the horizon and back synchronized with Primary Respiration and attunement to stillness as a therapeutic force. The fluid body also expresses the metabolic fields of the embryo when the practitioner is working within the tempo of Primary Respiration. These metabolic fields form the structures of the cranium discussed below. These fields are shaping processes mentioned in all of my books and especially the Glossary at the end of this volume.

- **The bones.** The next level of expression is the bones of the cranium, which are distinguished between the vault, the base, and the face. This is detailed in the photographs in this book. Cranial anatomy must be known, especially the types of sutures and beveling between cranial bones, for safe practice. Other distinctions at this level are made between interosseous motion and intraosseous motion. Each bone breathes with Primary Respiration by itself and then with each other. It is very easy to overfocus on the cranial bones and induce unnecessary compressions and side effects in the client when working mechanically for too long. The practitioner must broaden his or her attention regularly and join the cranial bones of the client with the entire osseous system of the client's body in the tempo of Primary Respiration. The biodynamic practitioner also learns how to sense the metabolic fields that built and maintain the cranial bones.

- **The meninges.** The next level of movement is the entire dural meningeal system as it expresses what is traditionally called flexion and extension. Another way of saying this from an embryonic point of view is folding and unfolding. Specific distinctions are made between the movement of the tentorium and the falx cerebri for proper evaluation of head injuries.

A description of this movement can be found in many books on craniosacral therapy. When the practitioner is able to concurrently maintain three dimensionality in himself or herself and the client, there is a different sensibility to this movement, especially in the tempo of Primary Respiration. This sensibility feels more like a global or systemic folding and unfolding of the whole shape of the body, not just the cranium. This is partially due to the continuity of the fascia of the meninges with the rest of the body fasciae and the metabolic fields that formed the fascia. As a note of importance, the meninges house most of the cranial nerves as they traverse the brain from the brain stem to their effector organs and it is very easy to irritate the meninges with mechanical techniques. This can induce entrapment neuropathies as described in the osteopathic literature.

- **The neural tissue of the brain.** The next level of movement is the neural tissue itself. Traditionally this is called flexion as the spinal cord moves superiorly and the cortex of the brain moves anteriorly and laterally in the shape of a ram's horn, according to Dr. Sutherland, followed by extension as the neural tissue reverses itself into extension. This also includes sensing the related motions of the cerebellum and brain stem in traumatized clients. These movements have important considerations in resolving all types of trauma, not just impact injuries to the head such as concussions. Concussions and their consequences must also be known in order to help clients whose history includes such trauma. Descriptions of these movements of the neural tissue can be found in many craniosacral therapy books.

- **Longitudinal and lateral fluctuations.** The *longitudinal* fluctuation is an expression of the *direct current* in the fluid body between the coccyx and the third ventricle mentioned throughout this book. It has a rate of two to three cycles per minute (CPM). It is the midline of the fluid body and does feel electric at times. The *lateral* fluctuation is paired with the longitudinal fluctuation and is a perpendicular bi-phasic vector of fluid movement to the median plane of the brain. The tempo and amplitude of the lateral fluctuation can also be an expression of stress in the fluid body, especially if it is experienced as speeding up or sensed as a figure-eight type movement that is also fast.

  Longitudinal and lateral fluctuations are specific faster potencies of Primary Respiration and exist in zone B and well as zone A. The practitioner must sense his or her own such potency in zone A and B related to the longitudinal and lateral fluctuations to access these potencies in the client. These are also referred to as Mid Tide potencies. Clinically, igniting the third ventricle is one way of helping the longitudinal fluctuation when it is weak.

- **Cerebrospinal fluid fluctuation.** The last level of motion that is distinguished is that of the cerebrospinal fluid. The CSF is an interstitial fluid that is connected to all the other interstitial fluids of the body. It is important to know its anatomy and physiology in relation to the meninges and cardiovascular system. Its movement patterns include circulation in the subarachnoid space, different kinds of fluctuations in each of the ventricles, and especially the third ventricle. The third ventricle is considered to be the apex of the biodynamic system.

This is just a brief tour of several different motions that a biodynamic practitioner may encounter while working on a client's head.

Appendix B

Recommended Reading in Visceral Manipulation

Barral, J., 2007. *Visceral Manipulation II,* revised edition. Seattle: Eastland Press.

This book goes into more detail on the major organs than the first volume (listed on the next page).

_____. 1991. *The Thorax.* Seattle: Eastland Press.

This book is very special, not only because of its anatomical detail, but also because it offers so many different skills for bringing freedom to the thorax.

_____. 1993. *Urogenital Manipulation.* Seattle: Eastland Press.

This is a very unique book detailing the precise anatomy and internal manipulation of the pelvic floor. While most licensed manual therapists are not able to perform intervaginal or interrectal manipulation, this book still serves a very important purpose in allowing the practitioner to understand the complexities of the pelvis, especially the need for some type of manipulation after surgery.

_____. 1996. *Manual Thermal Diagnosis.* Seattle: Eastland Press.

This book details Dr. Barral's method of diagnosing the viscera via the infrared heat given off by each organ. The hypothenar eminence at the base of the thumb has the greatest degree of sensitivity for perceiving these temperature variations.

_____. 2010. *Manual Therapy for the Prostate.* Berkeley, CA: North Atlantic Books.

This is an extremely important book for men and also details interrectal examination. It is valuable because men should be able to massage their own prostate gland on a regular basis. This book will show men how to do that.

Barral, J. and A. Croibier, 1999. *Trauma: An Osteopathic Approach.* Seattle: Eastland Press.
  This is an important book on working with the consequences of trauma on the organs and soft-tissue systems of the body. Of special interest are motor-vehicle accidents and high-velocity trauma, which would include mild traumatic brain injury or concussions.

_____. 2011. *Visceral Vascular Manipulations.* New York: Churchill Livingston Elsevier.
  This is one of the first books demonstrating how to work with the cardiovascular system in manual therapy.

Barral, J. and P. Mercier, 2005. *Visceral Manipulation,* revised ed. Seattle: Eastland Press.
  This is the revised edition of Dr. Barral's original book on the subject, with a special emphasis on his research on the kidneys.

Finet, G. and C. Williame, 2000. *Treating Visceral Dysfunction: An Osteopathic Approach to Understanding and Treating the Abdominal Organs.* Portland, OR: Stillness Press.
  This is one of the earlier books on visceral manipulation from the point of view of Belgian osteopaths. It is an important contribution to the field.

Hebgen, E. U., 2011. *Visceral Manipulation in Osteopathy.* New York: Thieme.
  I like this book a lot because it presents the theory and practice of several different experts in visceral manipulation. It also includes the circulatory techniques of Dr. Michael Kuchera, an American osteopath.

Helsmoortel, J., Hirth, T. and P. Wührl, 2010. *Visceral Osteopathy: The Peritoneal Organs.* Seattle: Eastland Press.
  This most recent book by Dr. Helsmoortel et al. is an important contribution to the expanding art and practice of visceral manipulation. The anatomy is superb and its orientation is very different orientation from that of the Barral books.

Keatley, M. and L. Whittemore, 2010. *Understanding Mild Traumatic Brain Injury (MTBI): An Insightful Guide to Symptoms, Treatments, and Redefining Recovery.* Boulder, CO: Brain Injury Hope Foundation.
  This is an important book detailing the consequences of concussions on the brain and body. It is important because the authors mention the effectiveness of craniosacral therapy in treating posttraumatic head and neck pain.

Kuchera, M. and W. Kuchera, 1994. *Osteopathic Considerations in Systemic Dysfunction.* Columbus, OH: Greyden Press.
  This is one of the only books I know of in the American osteopathic literature detailing work with the viscera and vascular system.

GLOSSARY OF BIODYNAMIC TERMINOLOGY

The glossary that follows this introduction is an attempt to describe fluidic perception. The focus is on the practitioner's somatic awareness. Consider this glossary as a tool for recognizing and locating one's place in the biodynamic therapeutic process. Biodynamic craniosacral therapy has evolved from three streams of important language, metaphor, and terminology. The first comes from the *palpation* skills developed by William Sutherland and subsequently his students. This is the language of describing what is happening in the client's body derived from information coming from the practitioner's hands. Sutherland was very fond of automotive and industrial metaphors in describing the inner workings of a client's body.

The second stream of terminology comes from the biodynamic embryology of Erich Blechschmidt and his interpreters, such as Brian Freeman and Jaap van der Wal. Biodynamic embryology developed a language based on the pure *observation* of the forces of growth and development in the human embryo. All science uses metaphors to describe newly observed phenomena such as the human embryo in the middle of the last century.

The third stream of language and metaphor comes from the field of interpersonal neurobiology (IPNB). The therapeutic relationship is described as a two-person biology. The basic language used in IPNB is about the therapeutic relationship as it is sensed in the practitioner's body, or simply *somatic awareness*. Thus IPNB is directly related to the philosophy of phenomenology of the body, in which the lived experience of the practitioner is the ground of observation and palpation. The term *lived experience* refers to a view that acknowledges the multidimensional aspects of our experiences, the context within which our experiences occur, and the meaning our experiences have in our lives. This includes our experience of space, time, our lived bodies, and our relationships. Our *lived bodies* allow us to perceive, interact with, and understand our world, and to make meaning of our experiences (Merleau-Ponty, 1962). Our bodily experiences, and the meaning they have in our lives, in turn shape our perceptions and future experiences with our body.

There are now other professions with unique language having impact on biodynamic practice. The disciplines of dance and movement therapy are of particular relevance in the creation of this glossary. In addition, in teaching I use terms from Jungian psychology, which includes language from mythology and shamanism. The rule of thumb is that a metaphor frequently involves an image. Sometimes the image is part of a story about a person's life. And finally, the story may be linked to a deeper origin mythology located in the unconscious. Certainly A. T. Still and W. G. Sutherland used religious and spiritual metaphors such as the "Breath of Life" and the "Master Mechanic," but I will save that part of the glossary for a later version. At this point in the evolution of the work, I prefer to use terms such as love, compassion, joy, and happiness as embodied sensation.

Consequently, I am making three different lists of terms and metaphors based on the above streams of information. I propose that these lists form an integrated whole for biodynamic perception and furthermore that this integrated whole perception was present in the osteopathic cranial concept from the beginning. The first listing includes the language of the biodynamic process. The second includes key terms regarding the bodily process of the practitioner. Finally, the third includes terminology associated with the interpersonal relationship of the practitioner and client.

The reader will notice that there is overlap between these categories, or what may seem to be redundancy. Biodynamic work is the work of wholeness and dissecting the whole into these parts is challenging at best, but necessary, because this terminology is used in classes constantly. It needs to have greater clarification regarding its meaning both as lived experience and secondarily as a theory or concept.

Biodynamic craniosacral therapy has evolved into a model of empathy and compassion, which is no longer simply a spiritual or philosophical construct, but rather a deeply embodied process resulting from the discovery of mirror neurons as well as other neurophysiological and cardiovascular research. This information has evolved into the discipline of interpersonal neurobiology, as mentioned above and throughout this volume. Therefore, the most fundamental principle in biodynamic practice is the somatic awareness of the practitioner. An important corollary to that is: when palpating the client always find the same place in the practitioner's body at the same time. All perception, mindfulness, and awareness arise from the whole body feeling sense of the practitioner. All of the terms and metaphors that follow need to be linked to direct lived experience in the body. Nothing is static in the body; it is all in process and, as Ann Wales, DO once said, the practitioner is putting hands on a horse that is already moving.

Please note: I do not use the word *energy* in this glossary because it means many different things to different people.

Practitioner Biodynamic Process (Fluid Perception and Self-Regulation Skills)

Orienting—Being quiet in body and mind, the practitioner is sensing her body three dimensionally. Shifting attention to fluid body buoyancy.

Synchronizing—Paying attention to Primary Respiration as it interchanges with stillness out through the zones and back. Relating Primary and secondary respiration together.

Attuning—Also *attunement*. The therapeutic skill of the practitioner moving his or her attention between self, the client, the office space, nature, and back in the tempo of Primary Respiration. Also the skill of not moving attention but rather recognizing and settling attention on Dynamic Stillness. Sometimes called *tracking* in other models of therapy. This approach to tracking is called *zone practice*.

Disengaging—The therapeutic skill of noticing when the autonomic nervous system settles and Primary Respiration becomes stronger.

Igniting—Also termed *ignition*. The therapeutic skill of noticing the strength and transition phases of Primary Respiration, and its interchange with Dynamic Stillness in any zone.

Bodily Processes (Shaping and Becoming)

Shaping—A form or the totality of one's biology whose three-dimensional contour is constantly changing from internal metabolic movement.

Body—An active shaping process mainly fluidic in nature. It is always in the living process of transforming and becoming something new. Sometimes referred to as *soma* or *somatic* or as the *organism* in some literature.

Embodiment—the ongoing process of the ebb and flow of body sensation free of judgment, projection, and interpretation (psychosomatic body). Related to the phenomenology of lived experience. Embodiment is always about the context of the body in space, time, and relationship.

Functioning—Sensing order and organization in the fluid body, which is the human body and the earth expressed as:

- Buoyancy, experienced as a lifting, floating, seaweed like movement
- Flow, the expressive and intentional direction of movement in the whole, also related to the quality of potency within an individual's fluid body

- Canalization or the appearance of fluid streams such as the longitudinal fluctuation from the coccyx to the third ventricle
- Integration and disintegration as gradients of density
- Assimilation (taking in) and dissimilation (eliminating waste products) in the fluids, related to different tempos or timing
- Spirals, twists, and turns
- Lateral fluctuations that are like three-dimensional figure eights

Potency—An expression of the ordering and organizing force of Primary Respiration permeating the fluid body. A feeling of three-dimensional amplification of Primary Respiration. Sometimes referred to as *health.*

Structuring—Growing and differentiating from cells to tissues to organs.

Metabolic fields—Activity of limiting (surface tension) tissue and inner tissues (watery and loose) in regards to all of the following:

- Specific position/location in the embryo (fluid body) such as a tight space or more open and thus the boundaries between fields are viscous and permeable
- Individual structure building via condensation or expansion of fluids or a combination of the two that have different densities and gradients
- Tempo (quiet/slow/fast) fluid movement in the embryo

    All metabolic fields in the embryo and adult body are characterized by order and organization. The whole of the fluid body is always taking shape by differentiating itself via metabolic fields in a way that is harmonious with what has come before.

Fluid body condensation—Expansion, including cell life and death, unfolds in the following sequence:

- Loosening
- Corrosion
- Suction
- Densation
- Contusion
- Distusion
- Retension

- Dilation
- Retraction

These sequential differentiations are defined below.[4]

Loosening—The watery element around inner limiting tissue that becomes the capillaries. This is seen in Figure G.1 as the water element expands naturally around the inner tissue of the embryo. The tailed arrow in the image shows the loss of fluid from cells. The number 1 indicates the expansion of intercellular substance between cells. The stipple shows the collective intracellular material.

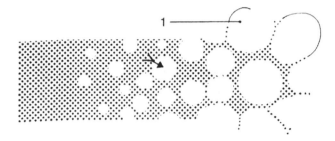

Figure G.1. Loosening fields

Corrosion—Dissolving boundaries so the two becomes one and flow can expand like the heart and kidneys. Cells die for connection to happen. Sense of hands melting into the surface of the body. This is seen in the stick Figure G.2. Boundaries dissolve because of the two tissues being so closely together that waste products and nutrition cannot enter that area and it dissolves.

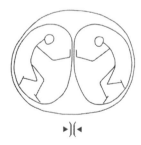

Figure G.2. Corrosion fields

4. The nine images here have been reprinted with permission from North Atlantic Books. They appear in *The Ontogenetic Basis of Human Anatomy: A Biodynamic Approach to Development from Conception to Birth* by Erich Blechschmidt, edited and translated by Brian Freeman. I have purposely left the distinguishing directional graphics beneath each image, which are not necessary for the understanding of this text, but for the ease of understanding of Blechschmidt's books, which I highly recommend.

Suction—The function of breathing locally and globally. Slow and fast tissues growing away from each other, sometimes pulling or tearing apart. This is seen in the image of a bellows with the stick Figure G.3.

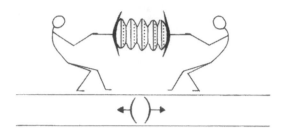

Figure G.3. Suction fields

Densation—Like squeezing a sponge that thickens into cartilage, with dehydration and thickening, beginning of skeletonization. It feels like torsion movements. This can be seen in the image of the stick Figure G.4.

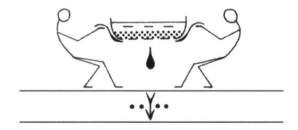

Figure G.4. Densation fields

Contusion—Compression of precartilage such as the whole spine around the surface of the body wall. Biomechanical compression. Cartilage appears first before muscles. This can be seen in the stick Figure G.5.

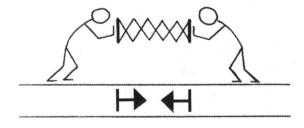

Figure G.5. Contusion fields

Distusion—Coupled with contusion. Expanding and growth swelling of cartilage on a midline axis (preferred direction). Occurs next to contusion fields pushing apart from each other. This can be seen in the stick Figure G.6.

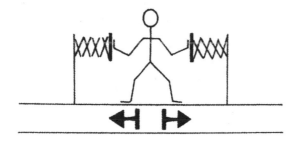

Figure G.6. Distusion fields

Retension—A taut rubber band. Growth resistance by bending and folding indicating a slow inner tissue and faster adjacent tissue. This is dynamic tension like on the notochordal midline, central part of the diaphragm. All tendons, ligaments, and joints form this way. Associated with Dynamic Stillness and natural quiescence in biological systems. Found in all the bends and folds of the embryo. This can be seen in the stick Figure G.7.

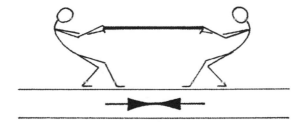

Figure G.7. Retension fields

Dilation—Coupled with retension, easily stretchable muscle building, expanding, and lengthening with torsion into available space such as the developing heart into the pericardium. Needs resistance of adjacent retension fields to form muscle at an acute angle to the retension field. May feel like sidebending of the tissue. This can be seen in the stick Figure G.8.

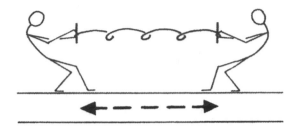

Figure G.8. Dilation fields

Detraction—Greater water loss, pulling apart, shearing, friction in glue-like substance. The way bones are made. This can be seen in the stick Figure G.9.

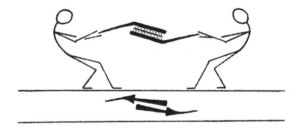

Figure G.9. Detraction fields

Symmetry—Organization around a fulcrum (such as umbilicus, heart, or third ventricle) or a midline (such as the spine). May occur asymmetrically, as with the limb buds. The arms use the fulcrum of the heart and the legs the fulcrum of the cloaca (anus).

Fulcrum—Point of organization in the early embryo associated with the kidneys (genitals), umbilicus (yolk sac), heart (chorion sac), and third ventricle (amnion sac).

Midline—Later organization of the embryo starting with the primitive streak and notochord and ending with the anterior midline.

Effort—Amount of potency the organism needs to complete a task against normal and above-normal resistance. Also *perseverance.*

Weight—Sense of gravity and its physical force drawing the body toward the earth.

Resistance—Experience of restriction from moving in a specific direction due to neighboring tissue or fluid gradients.

Imprinting—The four stages of morphology:

- Compression, usually associated with heat, condensation, and compaction
- Expansion, usually associated with a union or merging and deepening the relationship with the uterus
- Encapsis, pulling or tearing apart in order to form a middle, also associated with heart
- Folding/unfolding, the process of bending forward and backward, also growing up and down at the same time

Epigenesis—All factors influencing the expression of genes. This includes the effects of pre-conception and prenatal stress. Also the effects of the last meal ingested via the fluid body down to the cell nucleus.

Autonomic nervous system   The body's self-regulatory nervous system that manages breathing, digestion, heart rate, sexuality, and so on. Also related to the physiological defense mechanisms from stress. Another primary function is for conscious interoceptive awareness of body sensation and the regulation of joy and bliss.

Transforming—States of Primary Respiration and stillness.

Love—Longing to see others happy, as embodied and three-dimensional.

Joy—Personal experience of no self, embodied and three-dimensional.

Happiness—Well-being (freedom from suffering), embodied and three-dimensional.

Clarity and peace—The senses expand and open, embodied and three-dimensional.

Lighthearted—Able to lighten up and laugh, to release held tension, to forgive one's self and others, to see the meaning behind all of one's life events and story as it unfolded to the present moment. Thus able to live wholeheartedly.

Relational Processes (Empathy and Compassion)

Interpersonal neurobiology—Interpersonal nervous systems and cardiovascular systems.

Receptivity or empathy—Practitioner withdraws attention from hands periodically and notices the process by which the client is merging into practitioner's body via interoceptive awareness.

Interoception or cardioception—Conscious awareness of heart pulsation and movement of the blood and heart in the practitioner.

Intersubjectivity—Feeling felt by the other person as he or she also feels felt in the reciprocal therapeutic relationship of empathy.

Resonance—How practitioner focuses on personal somatic awareness to differentiate from client as both people are sharing or exchanging the same or similar bodily experience. The therapeutic skill is to not get lost in the client, or vice versa.

Insight or compassion—The therapeutic skill of knowing when to shift one's attention and hands.

Attuning—Practitioner moves attention deliberately and spontaneously back and forth through the zones. Called *tracking* in other therapies.

Circulating—Practitioner and client exchange roles as if in an embryonic state.

Perception—The purposeful or attentive consciousness of hearing, touching, seeing, smelling, tasting, orienting, and thinking.

Blood flow—Sense of heat being distributed in the body.

Hands and/or arms as umbilical cord—Sense of flow in the hands and arms.

Palpation skills—What the practitioner perceives or imagines sensing with his or her hands and body when in contact with the client.

Quietness—Natural state throughout the body as a result of growth resistance.

Confusion—Being fully present and self-regulated when in the natural state of not knowing. This is a regular occurrence in biodynamic practice.

Wholeness—Fluid body breathing as a single continuum in a three-dimensional sphere with Primary Respiration.

Neutral—Physiology of the autonomic nervous system disengages from high or low tone and settles. A sense of pooling or calm idling—settling into waiting.

Automatic shifting—Fluid body is free to change shape and be shifted or changed by the therapeutic forces of Primary Respiration after the neutral.

Normal—In biodynamic practice, a sense of buoyancy in three dimensions or simply floating or being lifted up through the core.

Health—Primary Respiration expresses itself more fully or powerfully. The amplitude and fullness of the potency of Primary Respiration is expressed.

Yielding—Dissolving of self, ideas, and mental chatter, and awareness of immersion into stillness.

Mindfulness—Moment to moment, nonjudgmental, nonreactive, present-time attention on an object of consciousness such as local breathing of Primary Respiration.

Awareness—Conscious interoceptive, panoramic attention that monitors the whole. Also called *central stillness* in biodynamic practice.

Mid Tide—A range of fluid tempos between one and four cycles per minute (CPM). One of these tempos is the longitudinal fluctuation.

CRI (cranial rhythmic impulses)—Fast tempos associated with a combustible autonomic nervous system.

Zones—Boundaries of awareness that dissolve into one thing, wholeness. The zones are:

- Zone A, the body;
- Zone B, the space around the body three dimensionally 15–20 inches off of the skin, also called the peripheral space in neurology associated with amygdala activity;
- Zone C, the office space as defined by the boundaries of the walls, the ceiling, and the floor; and
- Zone D, the natural world immediately outside the office all the way to the visible horizon or sky.

Natural world—The fluid body inside the skin and the world of nature outside the window as an interconnected whole with its own intelligence.

This glossary was reviewed and edited by Tim Shafer, Bill Harvey, and Carol Agneessens. Their touch and their minds have made the glossary much better. I am very grateful to Tim, Bill, and Carol for their help.

RESOURCES

Michael J. Shea, PhD
13878 Oleander Ave.
Juno Beach, FL 33408-1626
561.493.8080
www.michaelsheateaching.com
info@michaelsheateaching.com

Almut Althaus
Shea Educational Group European course administrator
Biodynamic craniosacral therapy practitioner
Shiatsu practitioner
Fohlenäckerweg 33
34130 Kassel, Germany
+49 (0)561 9885 0355
www.michaelsheateaching.de
althaus@movida-shiatsu.de

Sheila Shea, MA
Colon hydrotherapy instructor and practitioner
Raw food counselor
4427 East 5th St.
Tucson, AZ 85711
520.325.9686
www.sheilashea.com
intestines@sheilashea.com

Carol Agneessens, MS
Pacific School of Biodynamic Integration
Santa Cruz, CA
831.662.3057
www.holographictouch.com
carolagneessens@mac.com

Wendy Anne McCarty, PhD, RN
Prenatal and perinatal psychology practice for all ages, supporting
families and professionals, publications and information for individual
support available at www.wondrousbeginnings.com
315 Meigs Rd., A306
Santa Barbara, CA 93109
wmcarty@wondrousbeginnings.com

Sarajo Berman, MFA, CMT, LMT, RCST
Body therapist
2615 Cone Ave.
Durham, NC 27704
919.688.6428
sjberman@me.com

What Babies Want
Hana Peace Works
DVDs and books on birthing
P.O. Box 681
Los Olivos, CA 93441
www.whatbabieswant.com

Robert J Cutter, LAc, LMT
Acupuncture, bodywork, herbal remedies
55 Hitchcock Way, #105
Santa Barbara, CA 93110
805.698.0610
www.robertcutter.com

Claudine Laabs
Artist, photographer
561.655.9779
cleverglades@bellsouth.net

Sara Dochterman, LCSW
Psychotherapist
521 Lake Avenue, Suite 5
Lake Worth, FL 33460
561.533.0948
www.saradochterman.com
sara@saradochterman.com

Ann Diamond Weinstein, PhD
516.972.0388
adw@anndiamondweinstein.com

Castellino Prenatal and Birth Training
Contact: Sandra Castellino, MEd
1105 N. Ontare Rd.
Santa Barbara, CA 93105
805.687.2897
castellinotraining.com
sandra@castellinotraining.com

Tim Shafer, MS
Biodynamic craniosacral therapy instructor
3500 JFK Parkway, Suite 209
Ft. Collins, CO 80525
970.229.1925
www.indianpeaks.biz
Rolfer email: rolfer@indianpeaks.biz

Valerie A. Gora, LMT, BCST, NSCA-CPT
Biodynamic craniosacral therapy instructor
Continuing education in pre- and perinatal massage, infant massage,
and myofascial therapies
Excellent Bodywork, Inc.
North Palm Beach, FL 33408
561.283.3404
excellent-bodywork.com
valerie@excellent-bodywork.com

Pacific Distributing—Books and Bones
An extensive catalog in the fields of osteopathy, craniosacral therapy, embryology, anatomy, pre-and perinatal, neuroanatomy, physiology, somatic and trauma resolution, and movement therapies; carries some of the finest anatomical models in the world
Contact: Christopher or Mary Louise Muller
39582 Via Temprano
Murrieta, CA 92563
951.677.0652
www.booksandbones.com
booksandbones@verizon.net

Bill Harvey
Trainings and workshops in structural integration, biodynamic craniosacral therapy
3901 B Main St., 2nd floor
Philadelphia, PA 19127
215.681.1001
bill@billharvey.org

Esther Blessing
Praxis für Ganzheitliche Therapien
Biodynamic craniosacral therapy educator and practitioner
General Wille Str. 93
CH 8706 Feldmeilen
+41 (0)44 923 1001
Omirou Str. 6, Flat 202
1057 Nicosia, Cyprus
+35 (0)7 99 71 34 47

Marcel Bryner
Biodynamic craniosacral therapy educator and practitioner
Körpertherapeut
Wartstrasse 14
CH-8400 Winterthur
Switzerland
+41 (0)52 202 8477
marcel.bryner@bluewin.ch

Catherine Vitte
Biodynamic craniosacral therapy educator and practitioner
Asylstr. 119
8032 Zürich
Switzerland
+41 (0)44 383 33 34
www.vitte.ch

Biodynamic Craniosacral Therapy Association of North America
(BCTA/NA)
2501 Blue Ridge Rd., Suite 250
Raleigh, NC 27607
734.904.0546
www.craniosacraltherapy.org

BIBLIOGRAPHY

Abram, D. 1996. *The Spell of the Sensuous.* New York: Vintage Books.

Ainsworth, M. D. S., M. C. Blehar, E. Waters, and S. Wall. 1978. *Patterns of Attachment: A Psychological Study of the Strange Situation.* Hillsdale, NJ: Erlbaum.

Allan, C. B., and W. Lutz. 2000. *Life Without Bread: How a Low-Carbohydrate Diet Can Save Your Life.* Los Angeles: Keats Publishing.

Arumugam, M., J. Raes, E. Pelletier, D. Le Paslier, T. Yamada, D. R. Mende, G. R. Fernandes, J. Tap, T. Bruls, J. Batto, M. Bertalan, N. Borruel, F. Casellas, L. Fernandez, L. Gautier, T. Hansen, M. Hattori, T. Hayashi, M. Kleerebezem, K. Kurokawa, M. Leclerc, F. Levenez, C. Manichanh, H. B. Nielsen, T. Nielsen, N. Pons, J. Poulain, J. Qin, T. Sicheritz-Ponten, S. Tims, D. Torrents, E. Ugarte, E. G. Zoetendal, J. Wang, F. Guarner, O. Pedersen, W. M. de Vos, S. Brunak, J. Doré, MetaHIT Consortium (additional members), J. Weissenbach, S. D. Ehrlich, and P. Bork. 2011. Enterotypes of the human gut microbiome. *Nature* 473:174–180.

Atkins, R. C. 2002. *Dr. Atkins' New Diet Revolution.* Revised ed. Lanham, MD: M. Evans.

Audette, R. 2000. *Neanderthin.* New York: St. Martin's Press.

Barrows, S. 2001. The Great Yogurt (and Kefir) Conspiracy (cited June 20, 2011). Available from http://www.scdiet.net/healingcrow/HealingCrow/www.healingcrow.com/ferfun/conspiracy/conspiracy.html.

Barton, J., and J. Pretty. 2010. What is the best dose of nature and green exercise for improving mental health? A multi-study analysis. *Environmental Science and Technology* 44(10):3947–3955.

Basch, M. 1977. Developmental psychology and explanatory theory in psychoanalysis. *Annual of Psychoanalysis* 5:229–263.

Bates, E. 1979. *The Emergence of Symbols: Cognition and Communication in Infancy.* New York: Academic Press.

Beebe, B., S. Knoblauch, J. Rustin, and D. Sorter. 2005. *Forms of Intersubjectivity in Infant Research and Adult Treatment.* New York: Other Press.

Beebe, B., and F. Lachmann. 1994. Representations and internalization in infancy: Three principles of salience. *Psychoanalytic Psychology* 11:165.

Bentz, S., T. Pesch, L. Wolfram, C. de Vallière, K. Leucht, M. Fried, J. F. Coy, M. Hausmann, and G. Rogler. 2011. Lack of transketolase-like (TKTL) 1 aggravates murine experimental colitis. *American Journal of Physiology: Gastrointestinal and Liver Physiology* 300(4):G598–G607.

Bion, W. 1962. *Learning from Experience.* London: Karnac Books.

Blechschmidt, E. 2004. *The Ontogenetic Basis of Human Anatomy: A Biodynamic Approach to Development from Conception to Birth.* Berkeley, CA, North Atlantic Books.

Bradley, S. 2000. *Affect Regulation and the Development of Psychopathlogy.* New York: Guilford Press.

Brazelton, T. 1989. *The Earliest Relationship.* Reading, MA: Addison-Wesley.

Bremner, J. D., and M. Narayan. 1998. The effects of stress on memory and the hippocampus throughout the life cycle: Implications for childhood development and aging. *Development and Psychopathology* 10:871–888.

Briggs, J., and F. D. Peat. 1989. *Turbulent Mirror.* New York: Harper & Row.

Brunner, J. 1977. Early social interaction and language acquisition. In *Studies in Mother-Infant Interaction,* edited by H. R. Schaffer. New York: Norton.

Campbell-McBride, N. 2004. *Gut and Psychology Syndrome: Natural Treatment for Autism, Dyspraxia, A.D.D., Dyslexia, A.D.H.D., Depression, Schizophrenia.* Cambridge, UK: Medinform Publishing.

Chodron, P. 2011. Stay with your broken heart. *Tricycle,* Spring 2011, 16.

Coffey, D. S., and K. J. Pienta. 1991. Cellular harmonic information transfer through a tissue tensegrity matrix. *Medical Hypotheses* 34(1):88–95.

Coles, R. 1989. *The Call of Stories: Teaching and the Moral Imagination.* Boston: Houghton Mifflin.

Costerton, J. W. 2007. *The Biofilm Primer.* New York: Springer.

———, Z. Lewandowski, D. E. Caldwell, D. R. Korber, and H. M. Lappin-Scott. 1995. Microbial biofilms. *Annual Review of Microbiology* 49:711–745.

Crook, W. G. 1986. *The Yeast Connection: A Medical Breakthrough.* New York: Vintage Books.

D'Adamo, P. J. 1996. *Eat Right for Your Type: The Individualized Diet Solution to Staying Healthy, Living Longer & Achieving Your Ideal Weight.* New York: Putnam.

———, and C. Whitney. 2000. *Live Right for Your Type.* New York: Putnam.

Damasio, A. 1994. *Déscartes' Error: Emotion, Reason, and the Human Brain.* New York: Putnam.

———. 1999. *The Feeling of What Happens: Body and Emotion in the Making of Consciousness.* New York: Harcourt Brace.

de Wolff, M. S., and M. H. van Ijzendoorn. 1997. Sensitivity and attachment: A meta-analysis of parental antecedents of infant attachment. *Child Development* 68:571–591.

Demetrius, L. A., J. F. Coy, and J. A. Tuszynski. 2010. Cancer proliferation and therapy: The Warburg effect and quantum metabolism. *Theoretical Biology and Medical Modelling* 7(2).

Diez-Gonzalez, F., T. R. Callaway, M. G. Kizoulis, and B. Russell. 1998. Grain feeding and dissemination of acid-resistant Escherichia coli from cattle. *Science* 281:1666–1668.

Emde, R. N. 1989. The infant's relationship experience: Developmental and affective aspects. In *Relationship Disturbances in Early Childhood: A Developmental Approach,* edited by A. Sameroff and R. Emde. New York: Basic Books.

Emde, R. N., and J. E. Sorce. 1983. The rewards of infancy: Emotional availability and maternal referencing. In *Frontiers of Infant Psychiatry,* edited by J. D. Call, E. Galenson, and R. Tyson. New York: Basic Books.

Farah, H., and J. Buzby. 2005. U.S. Food Consumption Up 16 Percent Since 1970 (cited June 20, 2011). Available from www.ers.usda.gov/AmberWaves/November05/findings/usfoodconsumption.htm.

Field, T. 1985. Attachment as psychobiological attunement: Being on the same wavelength. In *The Psychobiology of Attachment and Separation,* edited by N. A. Fox. Orlando, FL: Academic Press.

Fonagy, P., M. Steele, H. Steele, G. S. Moran, and A. C. Higgitt. 1991. The capacity for understanding mental states: The reflective self in parent and child and its significance for security of attachment. *Infant Mental Health Journal* 12:201–218.

Fonagy, P., and M. Target. 1997. Attachment and reflective function: Their role in self-organization. *Development and Psychopathology* 9:679–700.

Gates, D., and L. Schatz. 2011. *The Body Ecology Diet: Recovering Your Health and Rebuilding Your Immunity.* Revised edition. Carlsbad, CA: Hay House.

Gergely, G., and J. S. Watson. 1996. The social biofeedback theory of parental affect-mirroring: The development of emotional self-awareness and self-control in infancy. *International Journal of Psychoanalysis* 77 (Pt. 6):1181–1212.

———. 1999. Early social-emotional development: Contingency, perception, and the social biofeedback model. In *Early Social Cognition,* edited by P. Rochat. Hillsdale, NJ: Erlbaum.

Gottschall, E. 2001. Elaine Gottschall: A Fountain of SCD Wisdom (cited June 20, 2011). Available from http://bit.ly/AjKnqC.

———. 2007. *Breaking the Vicious Cycle: Intestinal Health Through Diet.* Baltimore, Ontario, Canada: Kirkton Press.

Greene, E., and B. Goodrich-Dunn. 2004. *The Psychology of the Body.* Philadelphia: Lippincott Williams & Wilkins.

Haas, S. V., and M. P. Haas. 1951. *The Management of Celiac Disease.* Reprint. Philadelphia: J. B. Lippincott.

Haft, W. L., and A. Slade. 1989. Affect attunement and maternal attachment: A pilot study. *Infant Mental Health Journal* 10:157–172.

Heller, Rachael F., and Richard F. Heller. 1993. *The Carbohydrate Addict's Diet: The Lifelong Solution to Yo-Yo Dieting.* New York: Signet.

Hofer, M. A. 1984. Relationships as regulators: A psychobiologic perspective on bereavement. *Psychosomatic Medicine* 46:183-197.

———. 1994. Hidden regulators in attachment, separation, and loss. *Monographs of the Society for Research in Child Development* 59 (2–3, Serial No. 240):192–207.

Jaffe, J., B. Beebe, S. Feldstein, C. L. Crown, and M. D. Jasnow. 2001. Rhythms of dialogue in infancy: Coordinated timing in development. *Monographs of the Society of Research on Child Development* 66 (2, Serial No. 265):1–132.

Janet, P. 1929. *L'évolution psychologique de la personnalité.* Paris: Chahine. Reprint: Societé Pierre Janet, Paris, 1984.

Jealous, J. 1997. Healing and the natural world. Interview by Bonnie Harrigan. *Alternative Therapies* 3(1):69–76.

———. 2000. *Fluid Body 1.* CD Lecture Series.

Kabat-Zinn, J. 2005. *Coming to Our Senses: Healing Ourselves and the World Through Mindfulness.* New York: Hyperion.

Kennedy, D. P., J. Gläscher, J. M. Tyszka, and R. Adolphs. 2009. Personal space regulation by the human amygdala. *Nature Neuroscience* 12:1226–1227.

Kim, J., K. E. Peterson, K. S. Scanlon, G. M. Fitzmaurice, A. Must, E. Oken, S. L. Rifas-Shiman, J. W. Rich-Edwards, and M. W. Gillman. 2006. Trends in overweight from 1980 through 2001 among preschool-aged children enrolled in a health maintenance organization. *Obesity* 14(7):1107–1112.

Kirkengen, A. L. 2010. *The Lived Experienced of Violation: How Abused Children Become Unhealthy Adults.* Translated by E. S. Shaw. Bucharest: Zeta Books.

Klinnert, M. D., J. J. Campos, J. F. Sorce, R. N. Emde, and M. Svejda. 1983. Emotions as behavior regulators: Social referencing in infancy. In *Emotion, Theory, Research, and Experience,* edited by R. Plutchik and H. Kellerman. New York: Academic Press.

Krueger, D. 2002. *Integrating Body Self and Psychological Self: Creating a New Story in Psychoanalysis and Psychotherapy.* New York: Brunner-Routledge.

Lanius, R. A., P. C. Williamson, K. Bosksman, M. Densmore, M. Gupta, R. W. Neufeld, et al. 2002. Brain activation during script-driven imagery induced dissociative responses in PTSD: A functional magnetic resonance imaging investigation. *Biological Psychiatry* 52:305–311.

Lanyado, M. 2001. The symbolism of the story of Lot and his wife: The function of the "present relationship" and the non-interpretative aspects of the therapeutic relationship facilitating change. *Journal of Child Psychotherapy* 27:19–33.

Laplanche, J., and J. Pontalis. 1998. *The Language of Psychoanalysis.* London: Karnac Books.

Laszlo, E. 2009. *The Akashic Experience: Science and the Cosmic Memory Field.* Rochester, VT: Inner Traditions.

Levine, P. 2010. *In an Unspoken Voice: How the Body Releases Trauma and Restores Goodness.* Berkeley, CA: North Atlantic Books.

Lustig, R. Sugar: The Bitter Truth, July 30, 2009 (cited July 26, 2011). Available from www.youtube.com/watch?v=dBnniua6-oM.

Mahler, M. S., and M. Furer. 1968. *On Human Symbiosis and the Vicissitudes of Individuation.* New York: International Universities Press.

McConnell, H. 2001. Irritable Bowel Syndrome Patients Should Be Checked for Celiac Disease: A DG Review of: "Association of adult coeliac disease with irritable bowel syndrome: a case-control study in patients fulfilling ROME II criteria referred to secondary care," *Lancet* 358:1504–1508. P\S\L Group 2001 (cited June 20, 2011). Available from http://bit.ly/wbM4wl.

McEwen, B. 2002. *The End of Stress as We Know It.* Washington, DC: Joseph Henry Press.

McMillan, S. C. 2004. Assessing and managing opiate-induced constipation in adults with cancer. *Cancer Control* 11 (3 Supplemental 1):3–9.

McPartland, J. M., and E. Skinner. 2005. The biodynamic model of osteopathy in the cranial field. *Explore* 1(1):21–32.

Meaney, M. J. 2010. Epigenetics and the biological definition of gene-environment interactions. *Child Development* 81(1):41–79.

Merleau-Ponty, M. 1962. *The Phenomenology of Perception.* London, Routledge & Kegan Paul.

Nison, P. 2000. *The Raw Life: Becoming Natural in an Unnatural World.* New York: 343 Publishing Company.

Nocek, J. E. 1997. Bovine acidosis: Implications on laminitis. *Journal of Dairy Science* 80:1005–1028.

Ochs, E., and L. Capps. 1996. Narrating the self. *Annual Review of Anthropology* 25:19–43.

Ogden, P., K. Minton, and C. Pain. 2006. *Trauma and the Body: A Sensorimotor Approach to Psychotherapy.* New York: Norton.

Oh, M. S., K. R. Phelps, M. Traube, J. L. Barbosa-Salvador, C. Boxhill, and H. J. Caroll. 1979. D-lactic acidosis in a man with the short-bowel syndrome. *New England Journal of Medicine* 301:249–252.

Oppenheim, D., A. Nir, S. Warren, and R. N. Emde. 1997. Emotion regulation in mother-child narrative co-construction: Associations with children's narratives and adaptation. *Developmental Psychology* 33:284–294.

Ornish, D. 1995. *Dr. Dean Ornish's Program for Reversing Heart Disease: The Only System Scientifically Proven to Reverse Heart Disease Without Drugs or Surgery.* New York: Ivy Books.

Oschman, J. L. 2000. *Energy Medicine: The Scientific Basis.* Edinburgh: Churchill Livingstone.

Pally, R. 1999. *Mirror Neurons.* Los Angeles: Unpublished manuscript.

Patel-Thompson, J. 2006. *Listen to Your Gut: The Complete Natural Healing Program for IBS & IBD.* Revised, expanded edition. Vancouver: Caramal Publishing.

Persson, P. G., A. Ahlbom, and G. Hellers. 1992. Diet and inflammatory bowel disease: A case-control study. *Epidemiology* 3(1):47–52.

Porges, S. 2011. *The Polyvagal Theory: Neurophysiological Foundations of Emotions, Attachment, Communication, and Self-Regulation.* New York: Norton.

Rhoads, J. M., N. Y. Fatheree, J. Norori, Y. Liu, J. F. Lucke, J. E. Tyson, and M. J. Ferris. 2009. Altered fecal microflora and increased fecal calprotectin in infants with colic. *Journal of Pediatrics* 155(6):823–828.

Ridley, Charles. 2006. *Stillness: Biodynamic Cranial Practice and the Evolution of Consciousness.* Berkeley, CA: North Atlantic Books.

Rizzolatti, G., and M. Arbib. 1998. Language within our grasp. *Trends in Neuroscience* 21:188–194.

Rosen, M. E. 2008. Fluid (retrieved June 18, 2011). Available from www.osteodoc .com/fluid.htm.

Sander, L. 1975. Infant and caretaking environment: Investigation and conceptualization of adaptive behavior in a system of increasing complexity. In *Explorations in Child Psychiatry,* edited by E. J. Anthony. New York: Plenum Press.

———. 1977. The regulation of exchange in the infant-caretaker system and some aspects of the context-content relationship. In *Interaction, Conversation and the Development of Language,* edited by M. Lewis and L. A. Rosenblum. New York: Wiley.

———. 1995. Identity and the experience of specificity in a process of recognition. *Psychoanalytic Dialogues* 5:579–593.

Savino, F. P., L. Cordisco, V. Tarasco, E. Palumeri, R. Calabrese, R. Oggero, S. Roos, and D. Matteuzzi. 2010. Lactobacillus reuteri DSM 17938 in infantile colic: A randomized, double-blind, placebo-controlled trial. *Pediatrics* 126(3):e526–e533.

Savino, F. P., E. Pelle, E. Palumeri, R. Oggero, and R. Miniero. 2007. Lactobacillus reuteri (American Type Culture Collection Strain 55730) versus simethicone in the treatment of infantile colic: A prospective randomized study. *Pediatrics* 119(1), e124–e130.

Scaer, R. C. 2001. *The Body Bears the Burden: Trauma, Dissociation and Disease.* New York: Haworth Medical Press.

———. 2005. *The Trauma Spectrum: Hidden Wounds and Human Resiliency.* New York: Norton.

Scala, J. 2000. *The New Eating Right for a Bad Gut: The Complete Nutritional Guide to Ileitis, Colitis, Crohn's Disease, and Inflammatory Bowel Disease.* New York: Plume.

Schore, A. 1994. *Affect Regulation and the Origin of the Self: The Neurobiology of Emotional Development.* Mahwah, NJ: Erlbaum.

———. 2003a. *Affect Dysregulation and Disorders of the Self.* New York: Norton.

———. 2003b. *Affect Regulation and the Repair of the Self.* New York: Norton.

Shea, M. 2005. Class Notes.

———. 2008. *Biodynamic Craniosacral Therapy,* Volume Two. Berkeley, CA: North Atlantic Books.

Siegel, D. 1999. *The Developing Mind: Toward a Neurobiology of Interpersonal Experience.* New York: Guilford Press.

———. 2010. *Mindsight: The New Science of Personal Transformation.* New York: Bantam Books.

Smith, M. D. 2002. *Going Against the Grain.* New York: McGraw Hill.

———. 2003. *User's Guide to Preventing and Reversing Diabetes Naturally.* Laguna Beach, CA: Basic Health Publications.

Stern, D. N. 1971. A micro-analysis of mother-infant interaction: Behaviors regulating social contact between a mother and her three-and-a-half month-old twins. *Journal of American Academy of Child Psychiatry* 19:501–517.

———. 1977. *The First Relationship: Infant and Mother.* Cambridge, MA: Harvard University Press.

———. 1985. *The Interpersonal World of the Infant: A View from Psychoanalysis and Developmental Psychology.* New York: Basic Books.

———. 2000. *The Interpersonal World of the Infant: A View from Psychoanalysis and Developmental Psychology.* New York: Basic Books.

———. 2004. *The Present Moment in Psychotherapy and Everyday Life.* New York: Norton.

Stern, D. N., and J. Gibbon. 1978. Temporal expectancies of social behavior in mother-infant play. In *Origins of the infant's social responsiveness,* edited by E. B. Thoman. Hillsdale, NJ: Erlbaum.

Stern, D. N., L. Hofer, W. Haft, and J. Dore. 1984. Affect attunement: The sharing of feeling states between mother and infant by means of intermodal fluency. In *Social Perception in Infants,* edited by T. Field and N. Fox. Norwood, NJ: Ablex.

Taubes, G. 2011. Is Sugar Toxic? *New York Times Magazine,* April 13, 2011.

Trenev, N. 1998. *Probiotics: Nature's Internal Healers.* New York: Avery Trade.

Trevarthen, C. 1979. Communication and cooperation in early infancy: A description of primary intersubjectivity. In *Before Speech: The Beginning of Interpersonal Communication,* edited by M. Bullowa. New York: Cambridge University Press.

———. 1993. The self born in intersubjectivity: The psychology of an infant communicating. In *The Perceived Self: Ecological and Interpersonal Sources of Self-Knowledge,* edited by U. Neisser. New York: Cambridge University Press.

Tronick, E. Z. 1989. Emotions and emotional communication in infants. *American Psychologist* 44:112–119.

Tronick, E. Z., H. Als, and L. Adamson. 1979. Structure of early face-to-face communicative interactions. In *Before Speech: The Beginning of Interpersonal Communication,* edited by M. Bullowa. New York: Cambridge University Press.

Tronick, E. Z., H. Als, and T. B. Brazelton. 1977. The infant's capacity to regulate mutuality in face-to-face interactions. *Journal of Communication* 27:74–80.

Van der Kolk, B. A., and C. Ducey. 1989. The psychological processing of traumatic experience: Rorschach patterns in PTSD. *Journal of Traumatic Stress* 2:259–274.

Venes, D., ed. 2009. *Taber's Cyclopedic Medical Dictionary.* Twenty-first edition. Philadelphia: F. A. Davis Company.

Volokh, K. Y., O. Vilnay, and M. Belsky. 2002. Cell cytoskeleton and tensegrity. *Biorheology* 39(1–2):63–67.

Wadhwa, P. D. 2005. Psychoneuroendocrine processes in human pregnancy influence fetal development and health. *Psychoneuroendocrinology* 30:724–743.

———, L. Glynn, C. J. Hobel, T. J. Garite, M. Porto, A. Chicz-DeMet, A. K. Wiglesworth, and C. A. Sandman. 2002. Behavioral perinatology: Biobehavioral processes in human fetal development. *Regulatory Peptides* 108:149–157.

Ward, M. J., and E. A. Carlson. 1995. Associations among adult attachment representation, maternal sensitivity, and infant-mother attachment in a sample of adolescent mothers. *Child Development* 66:69–79.

Watson, J. S. 1994. Detection of self: The perfect algorithm. In *Self-Awareness in Animals and Humans: Developmental Perspectives,* edited by S. Parker, R. Mitchell, and M. Boccia. Cambridge, UK: Cambridge University Press.

Winnicott, D. W. 1990. *Home Is Where We Start From: Essays by a Psychoanalyst.* New York: Norton.

Wise, D., and R. Anderson. 2011. *A Headache in the Pelvis: A New Understanding and Treatment for Chronic Pelvic Pain Syndromes.* Occidental, CA: National Center for Pelvic Pain Research.

Wolf, N., M. Gales, E. Shane, and M. Shane. 2001. The developmental trajectory from amodal perception to empathy and communication: the role of mirror neurons in this process. *Psychoanalytic Inquiry* 21(1):94–112.

Wolfson, M. 2008. Carrageenan and the Acceptance of Food Additive Toxicity, 1950–2000 (cited June 20, 2011). Available from http://bit.ly/w1MaQv.

Xu, X., A. Z. Hausen, J. F. Coy, and M. Löchelt. 2009. Transketolase-like protein 1 (TKTL1) is required for rapid cell growth and full viability of human tumor cells. *International Journal of Cancer* 124(6):1330–1337.

Yudkin, J. 1978. *Sweet and Dangerous.* London: National Health Federation.

CLOSING THOUGHT

Since everything is but an apparition,
having nothing to do with good or bad,
acceptance or rejection, one may well
burst out in laughter.

Longchenpa (Tibet, 1308–1364)

ABOUT THE AUTHOR

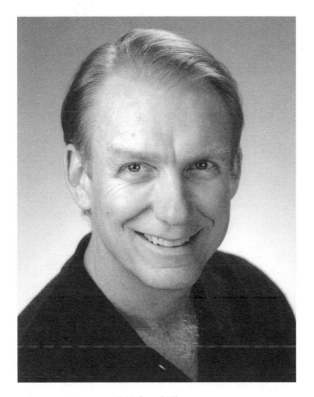

Michael Shea

One of the Upledger Institute's first certified Full Instructors of Craniosacral Therapy in 1986, Michael Shea, PhD, has taught somatic psychology, myofascial release, visceral manipulation, and craniosacral therapy worldwide for more than thirty years. He is cofounder of the International Affiliation of Biodynamic Trainings and a founding board member of the Biodynamic Craniosacral Therapy Association of North America. He is a student of His Holiness the Dalai Lama. Dr. Shea has also taught in the somatic psychology and pre-and perinatal doctoral programs at the Santa Barbara Graduate Institute and has served on several pre- and perinatal doctoral committees. He lives in Juno Beach, Florida, with his wife, Cathy. For more information on his courses and trainings, visit www.michaelsheateaching.com.